M000016705

The Cannabis Spa Book

Make Marijuana Lotion, Balm, Soak, Wraps, Bath Salts, Spa Nosh & More!

ISBN 13: 978-0615896526 (Hempista Press)
ISBN 10: 0615896529

Hempista Press ©2013 All rights reserved. No portion of this book, except for a brief review, may be copied or transmitted without permission. **www.hempista.com**

For spa lovers everywhere.

Contents

Chapters

PREFACE

This book is about the cannabis plant.

This book is about how to use cannabis to make you look and feel great, drawing from new and old traditions. It's a book about healing and elegance.

As of its first publishing date, in 2013, this book could get you in trouble if you happen to live in a location where the cannabis plant is still illegal. You may face a stint in jail, forced rehab and re-education, or even the death penalty for using the cannabis herb.

Because cannabis may be illegal in your location at the time of publication, this book is only recommended for those in locations where cannabis is legal for general or medicinal purposes. In some locations the speech in this book may be considered illegal as well. Please consult your local regulations or attorney for advice before purchasing this book or trying the recipes and techniques described herein.

Using the techniques and recipes in this book in locations where legal, tested and clean cannabis flowers and resins are not available, is not recommended.

Please consult your personal doctor for health information and diagnosis. This book is not intended to diagnose or treat any illness, and is not intended for pregnant or nursing mothers. Nothing in this book is approved by the FDA or any other government agency.

This book is intended for mature readers, 21 and older.

Why I Wrote This Book

I love our cannabis dispensary system in California. Our dispensaries have a wide selection of great edible products and brands, ranging from desserts, meals, drinks, and yes, body lotions and other topical cannabis products can be found in California dispensaries.

I was first introduced to topical cannabis products through a collective and I've been a huge fan of them ever since. I write about them on hempista.com, and I buy them frequently. I've purchased cannabis lip balms, lotions, creams, bath salts, and eye creams.

One of the most attractive features of external cannabis products is that they typically provide a way of medicating without the "high" that you get from vaporizing or ingesting cannabis orally. For me, this was a lifesaver for work time when I needed to be extra sharp, but still achieve pain killing results almost equivalent to a prescribed narcotic.

Like anything else, some of these I really liked and some were just so-so. Because the cannabis industry is still in its infancy, finding great cannabis products for external use can be challenging. One particular challenge for me is that the pain from autoimmune disease I suffer from can become vicious very quickly, and quite often the commercially available external cannabis products do not meet my needs. I also use topical cannabis preparations daily, and I need a fresh product that is free of preservatives and allergens.

So I started making lotions, bars, baths and everything in between, and in the process I discovered that this herb had so many useful applications for wellness, beyond the vaporizer or the brownie! It has become a daily part of my health & beauty regime.

I wrote this book as a way to share my private recipe book with others; these recipes have been refined and made as simple as possible so you can consistently reproduce my results at home.

For those who are beginners, I stick to mostly basic food-grade ingredients that are easy to find and work with. And for the advanced external preparations folks who would like to try out new techniques and materials for their repertoire, I've included some new techniques that are totally unique to this book and never written about before!

If you suffer from allergies or sensitivities this book is for you too! All the recipes in this book are free of allergens such as eggs, soy, tree nuts, peanuts, shellfish, yeast, mold, wheat, corn, gluten and dairy. *Please consult your doctor for allergy diagnosis and information on any of the ingredients if you are in doubt.*

Because this is a spa book, I've also included some of my favorite recipes for hemp smoothies and cannabis medicated beverages called "bhang". I also enjoy cannabis aromatherapy so I have included recipes for beautiful essence waters too.

There are so many ways to enjoy this beautiful herb, and it is my hope that you will find my recipes so useful that you will incorporate them into your wellness lifestyle.

An Introduction to Cannabis

Cannabis (/'kænəbɪs/; Cán-na-bis) is a genus of flowering plants in the family of Cannabaceae which includes Humulus (Hops) and Celtis (Hackberry). Within the Cannabis genus there are 3 primary variations, Cannabis sativa, Cannabis indica and Cannabis ruderalis. Cannabis is native to Asia and the first use of the plant for medicinal and general purposes is recorded there.

Cannabinoids

Cannabinoids are the active medicinal chemicals in the cannabis plant. Only one of these chemicals causes psychoactive effects, THC. There are 60+ cannabinoids in cannabis, including THC and CBD.

Aside from THC, the cannabinoid responsible for that "high" feeling when you vape or ingest cannabis, the plant may also contain a significant amount of CBD, a non-psychoactive cannabinoid that has many healing applications including pain relief, inflammation relief, and anxiety relief; CBD has also been shown to be effective in controlling seizures.

Consult your legal dispensary for strains that have been tested for cannabinoid levels, and then select the best strain for your needs based on this information.

Cannabis sativa is generally a tall and skinny plant with elongated leaves. This variety may be medicinally active or it may be the variety that is called "hemp," which is non-psychoactive and bred in particular for the seed and hurds, which can be made into many products. This form of Cannabis sativa, at the first publishing of this book, is legal to grow for these purposes in many places around the world including Canada, China and Europe.

When Cannabis sativa is grown for medicinal purposes the effects are heady and energetic. It can also be pain relieving as well, if it has a good percentage of naturally occurring CBD along with the THC. In my personal opinion, high CBD sativas provide the greatest amount of pain relief compared to any other strain - unless I want to sleep!

Cannabis indica is a short and broad leaf plant that can also express a range of purple, blue and pink colors.

Cannabis indica is always noted for its powerful cannabinoid content and has been used for thousands of years in Asia and the Middle East for making concentrated hashishes (50% or more THC).

Don't believe it at all if someone tells you "pot is stronger nowadays," it's simply not true! The powerful Cannabis indica plant has been used for thousands of years in concentrated form, much longer than prohibition has existed.

Cannabis indica has sleep inducing and narcotic properties which make it a great choice for evening pain control or relaxation. Naturally occurring CBD enhances the other qualities of the plant as well.

Cannabis ruderalis is a spindly and small plant without many of the qualities of the other two. Mostly, this variety is used for breeding purposes, to shorten the growing period for other variations. This variant isn't used in the recipes in this book unless it's part of the genetics of a hybrid variety.

Hybrid cannabis - Most cannabis is hybrid today. Although landrace strains remain a favorite with many connoisseurs, the hybrids have some interesting variations, flavors and colors that make them very popular.

Usually the hybrid will have most of the effects of the dominant strain; if there is more sativa than indica the hybrid might be a bit more heady and vice versa. A great hybrid is one that has a nice balance between the two. Not too sleepy, not too heady, and just the right amount of relief.

Hashish is traditionally made by shaking, extracting, or rolling the resinous trichomes from mature cannabis flowers grown for their medicinal qualities. This technique concentrates the cannabinoids into a crumbly powder or a resin ball.

Keif is made by gently shaking off trichomes from cannabis flowers grown for their medicinal purposes. It is fluffy and powdery. And although it is a concentrated form of cannabinoids, it tends to have less potency than hashish, but more potency than the whole dried flower.

Trim are the leaves trimmed from the buds before curing. These leaves contain the potent cannabinoids in smaller amounts than the flowers, and they're great for recipes where you don't really care about getting a lot of heavy green coloration from the chlorophyll.

Full-extract cannabis oil, **otherwise known as "Simpson Oil"** is a whole herb extract of cannabis oil that is made through an alcohol extraction process. This is an already decarboxylated cannabis product, unlike hashish, keif or cannabis flowers, and does not require heating to activate.

All of these forms of cannabis are used in the recipes in this book, and each recipe can be prepared with whatever form of cannabis you have available. The recipes are not strain-specific, so it's a good idea to select the strains that you find the most beneficial.

The Quick Start Guide

Get relief, right now, right from your cupboard!

In the process of putting together this guide, it occurred to me that successful pain and inflammation relief using a cannabis topical begins by learning simple techniques using ingredients that you have in your cupboard right now. Once you get comfortable with these techniques, the more complex recipes later in the book will help you explore new ways of working with and experiencing the cannabis herb.

Quick Start Ingredients

Olive oil is an ingredient most people have in the kitchen. It's also the one of the most effective fats for use with external cannabis preparations. Olive oils that are higher in oleic acid work best, delivering deep penetration of all the ingredients. Any kind of pure olive oil will work, but the kind that contains the highest amount of oleic acid is typically a fresh, cold pressed extra-virgin olive oil. High quality olive oils may have a cloudy appearance and a peppery taste.

Cinnamon (powder or stick), **ginger powder & cayenne pepper powder** are common spices found in many kitchens. They are noted for their warming and anti-inflammatory benefits and lovely, natural fragrance.

Salt is used in the bath and plunge recipes. I use a high quality, mineral rich ancient sea salt or Himalayan salt, but you can use Epsom, Kosher, or even plain salt that has <u>not</u> been enriched with iodine.

Cut lemons, **oranges, fresh mint & fresh ginger** are common fresh herbs that you may have in your kitchen right now. These will have cooling or warming properties depending on how they are used in the recipes.

Clean towels & **cloths** using any absorbent fabric, hemp or cotton is fine. You'll want a few sizes of towels and washcloths when doing the wraps.

Hot water, cold water, ice & heat packs are used with the wraps & soaks.

Cannabis in **trim**, **keif** or **ground flower** form is most effective for these recipes. You can make a highly effective and concentrated cannabis topical preparation using as little as 1/8 oz or 3.5 grams of ground flowers, or 1/2 oz or 14 grams of cannabis trim.

The less potent the cannabis, the more cannabis material you'll need to make an effective recipe. For example: if you are using a highly potent flower, perhaps 18% or more THC and/or 10% or more CBD, approximately 1/8 oz or 3.5 - 4 grams should be enough for each cup of olive oil. If you are using a lower potency flower, doubling the amount to 7 - 9 grams should work as well.

Quick Start Ointment Recipes

The Basic Quick Start Cannabis Ointment & Sensitive Skin Ointment

This recipe is specifically for more sensitive skin as it does not contain any of the supporting ingredients in the recipes that follow, such as cinnamon. This recipe has two ingredients only: olive oil and cannabis. This is the basic Quick Start Cannabis Ointment, and all of the other variations are based on this recipe.

You will need:

1 cup or 240 ml of olive oil

1/8 - 1/4 oz or 3.5 - 7 grams of ground cannabis flower including keif

OR

1 - 3 grams of keif

OR

1 cup oo/ '/2oz (handwritten)

1/2 oz or 14 grams of cannabis trim, chopped or ground

Preparation:

1.   Marinate cannabis in olive oil until saturated. Bake covered in a glass dish, in a preheated oven at 300 F or 150 C for 15 minutes. This process decarboxylates the cannabinoids.

2.   Allow this to cool and strain the oil from the plant material, squeezing as much of the oil out as possible. Set aside the plant material to use in the recipes that follow!

3.   Put the oil in a clean glass jar that has been sterilized in boiling water and dried.

TIP* You may use the oil immediately, but the best way to enjoy the benefits of this oil is to place it in the refrigerator and allow the oil to turn into a solid, semi-soft ointment which will be easy to apply and less "runny" compared to the oil at room temperature. It's also fantastically soothing to the skin; it has a cool and refreshing feeling as it melts upon contact.

After the oil has been refrigerated and has turned into a soft ointment, you will want to stir it after each use before refrigerating again. This will always ensure a creamy and smooth application each time.

Olive oil absorbs easily into the skin after several minutes, so you can feel free to apply as much as you would like while massaging into the skin. Or you can leave a thicker layer on the skin for applications such as the hot and cold towel wraps, or the soaks and baths recipes.

1 cup or 1 liter

Cinnamon Spiced Quick Start Cannabis Ointment

This recipe is just like the Basic Quick Start Cannabis Ointment, but with the addition of one of the most common and most medicinally effective spices in the kitchen: cinnamon. This oil is warming; the cinnamon and cannabis penetrate deeply into sore tissues and joints.

Take care not to get this preparation into open wounds or your eyes or mouth due to the heat from the cinnamon.

This recipe can be completed using either cinnamon sticks or powder.

You will need:

1 cup or 240 ml of olive oil

1/8 - 1/4 oz or 3.5 - 7 grams of ground cannabis flower including keif

OR

1 - 3 grams of keif

OR

1/2 oz or 14 grams of cannabis trim, chopped or ground

1 tsp or 2 grams of powdered cinnamon

OR

3 cinnamon sticks

Preparation:

1.   Marinate the cannabis and cinnamon in olive oil until saturated. Bake covered in a glass dish, in a

preheated oven at 300 F or 150 C for 15 minutes. Allow to cool.

2.   If you used cinnamon sticks, remove them first from the oil and set aside. Strain the plant material from the oil and set it aside for later use in other recipes.

Just like the Basic Quick Start Cannabis Ointment recipe, this formula is most effective when it is refrigerated and allowed to become a semi-soft ointment before application.

Healing Spice Trinity Quick Start Cannabis Ointment

This recipe incorporates three of the most common kitchen spices into a formula that is *very* warming and anti-inflammatory.

Like the Cinnamon Spiced Quick Start Cannabis Ointment, do not get this ointment in your eyes or other mucus membranes or any open wounds, because it is *very* warm.

You will need:

1 cup or 240 ml of olive oil

1/8 - 1/4 oz or 3.5 - 7 grams of ground cannabis flower including keif

OR

1 - 3 grams of keif

OR

1/2 oz or 14 grams of cannabis trim, chopped or ground

1 tsp or 2 grams powdered cinnamon

1 tbsp or 5 grams powdered ginger

1/2 tsp or 1 gram cayenne pepper powder

Preparation:

1.   Marinate cannabis, cinnamon, ginger and cayenne pepper in olive oil until saturated.

2.   Bake covered in a glass dish, in a preheated oven at 300 F or 150 C for 15 minutes. Allow to cool.

3.   Strain the plant material from the oil and set it aside to use with the poultice and wrap recipes. Stir the oil.

The oil is ready to use if you need pain relief right away! However, like the other versions of this recipe, this oil is best refrigerated first so that it turns into a semi-soft cold ointment.

Stir this oil after use and before refrigerating again for the best results.

Quick Start Hot & Cold Soaks & Baths

Hot, Tired, Swollen Feet? Take the Cool Plunge!

This foot plunge is like putting your feet into an ice cold mountain spring. This is very refreshing, and perhaps a little shocking. Your hot, tired and swollen feet will thank you!

There are some awesome foot soak recipes in the Getting High on Bath Salts chapter, so you'll want to check those out too once you've mastered this quick start foot plunge technique.

You will need:

Basic Quick Start Cannabis Ointment for Sensitive Skin

A foot spa soaker or basin

1/4 cup or 60 grams of salt

Cool to cold water to fill the spa or basin. Thoroughly dissolve the salt.

Optional but fabulous: juice from 1 fresh lemon & fresh mint that has been crushed a bit to release the essential oils directly into the water.

Preparation:

1.   Massage a generous amount of the cannabis ointment into your feet and ankles.

2.   Prepare your foot spa or basin with water and/or ice and lemon juice, then add the crushed mint leaves directly to the water.

After your feet have absorbed some of the oils from the cannabis ointment, about 15 minutes or so, you are ready to plunge them into the cold bath. Keep them there for as long as you like!

Painful Feet or Joints? Take the Warm Plunge!

This recipe can be used with either the Cinnamon Spiced Quick Start Ointment or the Healing Spice Trinity Quick Start Ointment. The latter will have more intensive warming effects.

You will need:

Cinnamon Spiced Quick Start Ointment or the Healing Spice Trinity Quick Start Ointment

A foot spa soaker or basin

1/4 cup or 60 grams of salt

Warm to hot-as-you-can-stand-it water to fill the spa or basin. Be sure to thoroughly dissolve the salt.

Optional but fabulous: juice from 1 fresh lemon & 1 large ginger root sliced and added directly to the hot water.

Preparation:

1.   Massage a generous amount of the cannabis ointment into your feet and ankles.

2.   Prepare your foot spa or basin with the heated water and the salt, then add the lemon juice and sliced ginger to the heated water.

After your feet have absorbed some of the oils from the cannabis ointment, about 15 minutes or so, you are ready to plunge them into the warm foot bath.

Cool Off Now: The Full Body Fever Plunge

This is great for sunburn, fever or any time you need to cool down right away.

You will need:

Basic Quick Start Cannabis Ointment for Sensitive Skin

A tub filled with cool water

A blender

1/2 cup or 125 grams of salt

2 large sliced oranges

1 large bunch of fresh mint

2 cups or 480 ml of hot water

Preparation:

1.   Fill the bath with the salt and the coolest water temperature that is most comfortable for you.

2.   In a blender combine the hot water, mint leaves and oranges. Blend until chopped, but not smooth, because you will want to strain this bath tea, especially if you are using a jet tub for your plunge. Strain the resulting tea and add to the bath water.

3.   Generously apply the cannabis ointment to the heated areas of your body that need to cool down. Allow this to soak in for about 15 minutes before plunging into the bath.

Warm Up Now: The Full Body Hot Plunge

This is my favorite quick start bath when I hurt, literally everywhere. You'll want to adjust the temperature of this bath to be as hot as possible for the maximum benefit.

You can use any of the ointment recipes, but the best results are obtained with either the Cinnamon Spiced Quick Start Cannabis Ointment or the Healing Spice Trinity Quick Start Cannabis Ointment.

You will need:

The Quick Start Cannabis Ointment of your choice

A tub filled with warm to hot-as-you-can-stand-it water

A blender

1/2 cup or 125 grams of salt

1 cut lemon

1 large sliced ginger root or 1 tbsp or 5 grams of ginger powder to substitute

2 cups or 480 ml of hot water

Preparation:

1.   Generously apply the cannabis ointment to all areas that need relief. While this penetrates into your skin for 15 minutes, prepare the bath water with salt.

2.   In a blender coarsely blend the ginger, whole lemon and hot water. Strain the tea and add to your bath. Plunge into your bath immediately!

Painful Hands? Try the Quick Start Warm Hand Plunge!

Do you have arthritic or otherwise painful hands? Your hands will feel better within minutes using this warm hand plunge.

This recipe works the best with the Cinnamon Spiced Quick Start Cannabis Ointment or the Healing Spice Trinity Quick Start Cannabis Ointment, and can be done in your sink.

You will need:

The Quick Start Cannabis Ointment of your choice

1 sink or basin full of warm to hot-as-you-can-stand-it water

1/4 cup or 60 grams of salt

1 large sliced ginger root or 1 tbsp or 5 grams of ginger powder to substitute

Preparation:

1.   Massage the ointment into your hands and allow 15 minutes to penetrate into the skin.

2.   Prepare your sink or basin with warm to hot water and salt. Add the sliced ginger root and agitate. Plunge!

Quick Start Wraps & Poultices

Wraps and poultices are a fast and intensive method of using cannabis topically. Many folk medicine practices include the use of wraps and poultices precisely because they are so effective for applications such as pain relief. Traditional medicinal use of cannabis in Asia almost always included the topical application of the leaves.

Some of these recipes utilize the plant material leftovers from making the quick start ointments. Please note that that leftover trim or flower from the ointments that contain warming spices may irritate rashes and shouldn't be used on any open wounds.

Quick Start Simple Cannabis Wrap – Hot or Cold, Your Choice!

If you are experiencing heat and inflammation cool down with a moist, cooling wrap that uses the Basic Quick Start

Cannabis Ointment.

You will need:

Basic Quick Start Cannabis Ointment for Sensitive Skin

3 - 4 clean towels

1 large pan or basin of ice water, including ice chips or cubes

Optional: add crushed mint leaves to the cold water

Preparation:

1.   Generously apply the cannabis ointment to the affected area.

2.   Soak one towel in the ice water and squeeze. Wrap the cold towel around the area that you have applied the cannabis ointment to for 15 - 20 minutes.

If needed, cool the towel again in the ice water and reapply. For more intensive relief, ice packed inside of 2 cool, moist towels wrapped around the affected area is suggested.

Brewing mint tea or crushing mint leaves in the ice water will add an additional cooling sensation to this wrap.

For the Hot Wrap

You will need:

Any of the quick start ointments will work, but for best results use the Cinnamon Spiced Quick Start Cannabis Ointment or the Healing Spice Trinity Quick Start Cannabis Ointment

3 - 4 clean towels

1 large pan or basin of hot water and/or hot packs or a moist heating pad

Preparation:

1.   Apply the ointment generously to the desired areas. If you using hot water only, dip one towel in the water, squeeze and apply immediately. Wrap an additional dry towel around the warm, wet towel. This should continue to produce heat for 15 - 20 minutes.

2.   If you have heat packs or a heating pad, prepare a warm, moist towel the same way and wrap the area placing the hot pack or heating pad on top of the warm, moist towel. Wrap this with a dry towel. This will be effective when you need heat for 30 minutes or more, or a more intensive heat overall.

Quick Start Cooling Cannabis Poultice

Poultices have long been a part of traditional medicine across many cultures. Typically these preparations consist of ground or macerated herbs, clays and resins that are applied directly to the skin. For example, fresh cannabis leaves were applied directly to the skin as a poultice in some ancient texts from India.

This cooling poultice contains cannabis and some common kitchen herbs, and uses the leftover plant material from making the Basic Quick Start Cannabis Ointment, which contains no added warming spices.

You will need:

The leftover cannabis flower or trim material from making the Basic Quick Start Cannabis Ointment

1 tbsp or 15 ml of cold water

1 bunch of fresh mint leaves

A few ice chips to cool the mix

A blender

Clean wrapping gauze

Preparation:

1.   Put the cannabis material, mint leaves and water into the blender and blend until smooth. Add an ice chip and blend again briefly to cool the mixture down.

2.   Apply this paste to the desired area and wrap with clean gauze. Apply additional ice packs or other moist cooling wraps as needed.

TIP* This recipe also makes a great forehead compress. Prepare the mixture as you would to wrap, but instead apply to the forehead and temple area and use a cold washcloth or compress over the area.

Quick Start Warming Cannabis Poultice

My favorite way to use this poultice is on my arthritic hands, which are then covered with spa gloves that I've warmed in the dryer. It's also great for achy joints and muscles and can even be combined with head packs or wraps.

You will need:

The leftover cannabis flower or trim material from making any of the quick start ointments (The Cinnamon Spiced Quick Start Cannabis Ointment or the Healing Spice Trinity Quick Start Cannabis Ointment leftovers will have the greatest warming effect.)

1 large sliced ginger root or 2 tbsp or 10 grams of ginger powder to substitute

3 tbsp or 45 ml of boiling water

A blender

Clean wrapping gauze

Preparation:

1.   Put the cannabis material, ginger and boiling water into the blender and blend until it is a smooth paste.

2.   Apply this mixture to the desired area and wrap with clean gauze. Apply additional moist heat as needed.

Chapter 1: The Basics - Materials and Methods

In this chapter, you'll learn about the ingredients and techniques used to make the most simple to the most luxurious cannabis topical preparations.

I am a home herbalist who has been making my own external cannabis products to treat the sometimes unrelenting pain of autoimmune disease and deal with the side effects of the life-saving drugs and treatments I've had.

Because of my condition, I've taught myself to make external cannabis preparations with ingredients that are free of artificial colors, flavors, fragrances and preservatives. This makes these preparations as allergen-free and immune system friendly as possible.

Most external cannabis preparations will not cause any psychoactive effect and provide local relief only. For intensive pain relief, external cannabis products may be combined with vaporized or ingested cannabis.

The recipes in this book are based on simple food-grade ingredient formulas, basic kitchen techniques, and (mostly) easy to obtain ingredients, so you can learn the art of making cannabis spa and wellness products quickly and without the headaches of mistake batches.

It's important to follow the recipes and not substitute ingredients when you are starting out, as mistake batches can be difficult to reclaim. However, as you begin to understand the principles, and become familiar working with the preparations, you can add some of your own creative ideas to the mix!

The great news is that it's easier and more budget friendly than you may think to make very effective and high quality external cannabis preparations in your own kitchen.

The Small Batch Philosophy

These are small batch recipes. External cannabis products work better and are much fresher when made in small batches that are used quickly. You may double or triple any recipe, but for the purposes of the home cook who makes these recipes for only one or two people, small batches are the best way to minimize waste and have a fresh product on hand at all times.

In the Quick Start chapter, you have already learned how to make simple cannabis ointments with just a few ingredients using refrigeration. That instruction is similar to the rest of the recipes in the book.

Most spa recipes in this book are perishable because they contain food-grade ingredients. You'll be creating small batches of cannabis spa products every few weeks, which should be refrigerated in most cases.

Most spa products that are shelf stable must contain a preservative to prevent microbial growth. This is why the recipes in this book use small batches, refrigeration and quick use within 30 - 60 days as a rule of thumb.

I don't use preservatives and I do not recommend them. Remember: antioxidants like vitamin E are not preservatives and will not prevent microbial growth.

You won't believe how fabulous it feels to use a lotion or scrub right out of the fridge. This is so refreshing and simple you will say "ahhhhhh!" Fresh, simple ingredients are not only luxurious, but good for you too.

Oils, Herbs, Resins, Water, Waxes, Weed, Oh My!

It's wise to assemble a kit in which you can organize all of your spa-making supplies. Most of the supplies you will need can be found in your own kitchen. There are a few you may need to obtain at a local Asian or ethnic grocery, natural grocer, or online. At the end of this book you will find a resources section which will help you obtain some of the more exotic ingredients used in some of the recipes.

Many of the ingredients in the recipes here are common in central Asian cuisine and wellness preparations. Cannabis is also native to this area, so it is not surprising that the first medicinal cannabis traditions for topical applications originated in the herbal apothecary of central and south Asia. Cannabis has a wonderful synergy with the herbs and spices originating from this region of the world.

The following ingredients constitute the basic cannabis spa-making supply kit you'll need in order to start making all of the recipes in this book. Feel free to add to your kit as you discover new fragrances and herbs!

It's my hope that, along with discovering new ways to experience wellness and joy with cannabis, you'll also discover the pleasure of using other herbs as well.

Base Fats High in Oleic Acid

The recipes in this book utilize base fats high in oleic acid because oleic acid is much more efficient at delivering cannabinoids transdermally compared to any other kind of fatty acid. Fats high in oleic acid also absorb better into the skin, leaving less to make the skin sticky or oily.

Olive oil that is fresh and cold pressed is best, the more fresh and virgin the olive oil, the higher oleic acid content; this is what you need to deeply penetrate into the skin. Olive oil is also an excellent skin softener.

Sunflower oil is another oil which is high in oleic acid and an excellent emollient. I use this oil in many of the recipes where the greenish color of olive may not work well.

Mango seed butter is a softer seed butter high in oleic acid that comes from the seed of the mango fruit. It absorbs well into the skin and is a great substitute for shea butter, which may cause sensitivity in those allergic to latex.

Cocoa butter comes from the cocoa bean and smells like a yummy chocolate bar! This butter is used in the Tropical Paradise Tanning Bar recipe. Cocoa butter is one of my all time favorite oils to tan with because of its scent and beneficial emollient properties. It's also higher in oleic acid.

Tucuma & murumuru palm butter come from palm trees that provide a seed which produces a solid butter high in oleic acid. This butter has a slightly "soapy" fresh essence that works well with florals like rose. These butters are used in the lotion bar recipes.

Dry Ingredients

Sapindus Mukorossi is also known as the soap nut or soapberry, and is a Himalayan treasure that is the centerpiece of the emulsion technique you will learn for creating cannabis baths, soaks and washes. The soapberry emulsifies all oils and distributes them in the water so they do not float on the surface, but rather penetrate deeply into your skin. The soapberry is superior because it is a low-foaming saponin, which makes it perfect for jet baths and other bath and soak applications. Sapindus Mukorossi has been used for thousands of years in Ayurveda (the traditional medicine of India) for skin and hair health, and complements the cannabis herb perfectly.

Here in the west people normally use the soapberry for laundry purposes. They are commonly found in the laundry section of most natural food stores. Soapberries, aside from their presence in the cannabis spa techniques in this book, make a superior all-around great household soap for those with allergies, skin conditions or other special health needs. They are non-drying, anti-inflammatory and anti-microbial. You don't need to wear gloves while cleaning your home with soapberries! The herbal water filled with saponins is good for your hands and the environment.

At the end of this chapter you will find recipes that are great for general cleaning and also disinfecting, using the authentic Sapindus Mukorossi soapberry.

Pink Himalayan sea salt *or any other sea salt* - I like ancient salts the best for their fabulous mineral profile, which creates a very healing bathing experience.

Citrus peels fresh and dried. You'll need lemon peels to make the basic bath recipes, and orange peels for fragrance in some of the bath salts. Some of the recipes call for blood orange peels, but you may substitute these with regular orange peels. Blood orange peels have the fragrance of orange with a slight note of berry and add a pink or reddish color to the recipes.

Spice mix - The recipes use an assortment of spices and herbs to impart fragrance and healing qualities. Whole spices are recommended for best results: Cinnamon Sticks, Cardamom Pods, Cloves, Star Anise, Turmeric Root, Black Tea, White Tea, Roses, Ginger Root.

Fresh flowers and herbs - Be sure to have some roses, citrus leaves and flowers, garden herbs, mints and other fragrant herbs and flowers on hand!

Essential Oils

Essential oils - Pick your favorite! Luxury ingredients are used in some of the recipes here, like floral attars, but you can use any of your favorite essential oils with these recipes: Jasmine, Rose, Ylang Ylang, Lavender, Peppermint, Rosemary, Ginger, Lemon, Amber Resin, Henna Flower Attar.

Sunflower lecithin is an essential ingredient for creating the emulsions that will become lotions, creams and other preparations. It is free of GMO and industrial extractions. I purchase sunflower lecithin in a capsule form that can be broken open and the lecithin squeezed out. This is very convenient when measuring out lecithin in the recipes because the capsules are already in a 1 gram pre-measured size.

Waxes

Floral wax is the naturally occurring wax in some flowers and is the product of essential oil extraction. Floral waxes smell like their respective, and much more costly, essential oil cousins like Rose Otto, Jasmine Sambac, etc. These waxes are vegan and are used for making many of these recipes in place of beeswax. The scent is light and natural.

Beeswax can be used in place of the floral waxes in any of the recipes that call for floral wax. I use it in some topical products, and it contributes a lovely fragrance profile you just can't get anywhere else, if you decide to use it as a substitute for the floral waxes called for in the recipes.

If you have allergies be aware that beeswax may contain some pollen and fungus, depending on the quality of filtration.

Floral Waters, Hydrosols and Aloe Vera

Floral Water "Hydrosols" - You can get these at an ethnic grocery, natural store or online. They are a product of a process that uses steam distillation to extract the essential oils. They come in fragrances like rose, neroli and mint. You'll see these most frequently as "rose water", "orange flower water", "orris root water" and "mint water" in retail bottle packaging; they are intended as flavorings for food and drink.

These culinary flower waters are food-grade and contain only citric acid in addition to the distilled floral water. They do not, and should not contain preservatives, and need to be kept refrigerated after they are opened.

Additionally, you can make essence water, which performs functionally like the commercial hydrosol, but is made through another process which is discussed in Chapter 5. Essence waters are not distilled and have a very short refrigerated life. They are best used immediately - within 3 days in any recipe or other use.

Aloe vera is used frequently in the recipes in this book. I almost exclusively use fresh aloe vera gel directly from fresh harvested leaves. You may use a commercial gel or liquid that is preservative-free. Aloe may be a bit "chunky" when it is scraped fresh from the leaves, but in these recipes it is blended smoothly in a blender before adding to lotions or other preparations.

Everything Else

Sanitizing products - My simple Soapberry Thieves recipe is great for sanitizing your counters and cooking equipment, and brewer's iodine is best for sanitizing containers. The potential for microbial contamination in spa products is as great, if not greater, than in food products.

You'll want to sanitize all containers and working surfaces before starting your work.

Assorted glassware, glass bowls, a warming and cooking pan, and wooden utensils - Use these to make and store your cannabis products.

Cannabinoid Containing Materials

Clean, finely ground cannabis flowers - These are a must-have. Even if you don't have access to more concentrated cannabis products, you can make any of these recipes using cannabis flowers. Trim is not used in any of the topical recipes, however trim can be used with the bath recipe in Chapter 3.

Full-Extract Cannabis Oil also known as **"Simpson Oil"** - Popularized by cancer survivor Rick Simpson, this unique oil is fully decarboxylated and ready for use. No need to cook or heat this oil. Available at legal dispensaries, or check out his recipe on his web site: phoenixtears.ca .

Simpson oil will stain your skin slightly green from the chlorophyll when it is used in a topical preparation, so you may not want to use this oil in preparations where you need to avoid staining skin or clothing.

This is a whole food extract of cannabis made using alcohol, which is then evaporated away through a cooking process. The resulting oil contains all of the plant properties including chlorophyll. Simpson oil is best for topical applications that call for intensive medicinal benefits - green stains and all!

Keif or Hashish - A raw concentrated cannabis product, like ground flowers, that has not been decarboxylated. This is the best for creating cannabis oils with little or no green coloration. Keif is more fluffy and light, while hashishes are more concentrated and sticky.

Working with Cannabis

Before you can begin making these products you'll need to start with cannabis bases that are fat based. This is important because the cannabinoids in cannabis are not water soluble, and require fats or alcohol to dissolve.

The recipes in this book utilize the technique of decarboxylation, which is the same technique used in cannabis food products. Decarboxylation is the process of shedding a carbon atom from a carbon chain when cannabinoids are heated to the appropriate temperature - approximately 250 - 300 F or 135 - 150 C for 15 - 30 minutes. If this sounds complicated, it's not. Basic cooking skills are all that is required to make a really effective cannabis spa product.

The "Does Everything" Cannabis Foundation Oil

You will be making a fully decarboxylated cannabis oil in an oil base that is high in oleic acids. This "foundation oil" will work in any recipe, and is the foundation upon which the other recipe ingredients are built.

The only spa recipes in this book that do not use the foundation oil are the bath recipes, which use their own cannabis oil technique during the cooking process.

Cannabis Flower Foundation Oil

You will need:

1/2 oz or 14 grams of finely ground cannabis flowers. Strains rich in cannabinoids work the best. Select your favorite strain with the qualities that appeal to you the most when making this foundation oil. Double this amount for strains lower in cannabinoids.

1 cup or 240 ml olive or sunflower oil

Preparation:

1.   Fully saturate the ground cannabis in the oil and let it sit overnight before baking in a covered glass dish in an oven that has been preheated to 300 F or 150 C for 15 minutes.

2.   Set aside to cool and then strain and squeeze as much oil as you can from the material. Refrigerate this oil immediately.

3.   Set aside the strained cannabis maceration for a second process that is used in the salt scrub recipes, poultices, and mud mask.

Or, you may process the maceration a second time by marinating in oil again for several days on the counter. The second process will be much lower in cannabinoids.

Keif or Hashish Foundation Oil

Keif is my favorite form of raw cannabis when making foundation oil because of its versatility. Keif retains a lot of the same fragrance profile as the ground flower if it has been kept tightly sealed. These additional flavonoids and terpenes are potent helpers alongside the cannabinoids.

Keif or hashish is more powerful than the ground cannabis flower foundation oil, because it contains more cannabinoids and less plant material.

The basic recipe calls for 6 grams of keif or hashish. You may use less or more, but in my test kitchen, 6 grams was the most effective for making very cannabinoid-rich topical products.

The other advantage of using keif or hashish is that the final foundation oil product ends up being less green than products made with cannabis flowers. The tanning bars, for example, call for blonde keif; the more blonde or lightly colored your concentrated cannabis product, the lighter the oil will be.

You will need:

6 - 10 grams of keif or hashish

1 cup or 240 ml olive or sunflower oil

Preparation:

1.   Fully saturate the keif or hashish in the oil and let it sit overnight before baking in a covered glass dish in an oven that has been preheated to 300 F or 150 C for 15 minutes.

Set aside to cool. Strain the oil if necessary and refrigerate immediately.

Full-Extract Cannabis Oil (Simpson or RSO) Foundation Oil

Making a foundation oil for use with these recipes is simple and requires no additional heating if you use full-extract cannabis oil (otherwise known as Simpson Oil or RSO). This product contains a significant amount of chlorophyll and may impart a slight green tint to your skin, which is why this oil is best used in recovery and healing applications, as in the traditional "Kaneh Bosem" recipe.

You will need:

6 - 10 grams of full-extract cannabis oil

1 cup or 240 ml of olive or sunflower oil

Preparation:

Fully dissolve the tar-like full cannabis extract oil into the base oil. Refrigerate.

I'm a Soapberry Evangelist, and You Should be Too!

You've already read about the soapberry (Sapindus Mukorossi) earlier in this chapter, and the ways it can be used for sanitizing your working area as well as for emulsification applications in the other recipes that follow in later chapters.

Soapberries can perform every job - and quite well I might add - that any commercially prepared soap, shampoo, detergent or cleaner can tackle.

If you are trying to avoid preservatives it is important to remember that all liquid soaps and cleaners, regardless of the organic labelling, must contain a preservative to prevent spoilage. Soapberries are dried and activated with water later, so they never require a preservative.

Basic Soapberry Liquid for Hair & Skin

Skin sensitivities and allergies? This soapberry preparation is simple to make and very refreshing.

Soapberry liquid is naturally low-foaming, which may take some time to adjust to, if you are fond of the mountains of foam that many commercial shampoos and soaps produce. Strained through muslin or a coffee filter, this liquid soap will work great in a foam dispenser bottle and actually foams quite nicely.

Soapberries have an earthy, cooked pineapple or vinegar fragrance. I add a few citrus peels (lemon or orange) to the liquid, along with a drop or two of essential oil.

You will need:

50 Sapindus Mukorossi soapberries, seeded and split in half

2 cups or 480 ml water

Optional:

A few citrus peels dried or fresh

Any essential oil of your choice

TIP* Some people like to use cannabis in this recipe for relief from various skin conditions. Doing this is simple: add 1 gram of finely ground cannabis flowers.

Preparation:

1.   Briefly rinse the dry soapberries in a strainer and add to a bowl. Add a few citrus peels and/or cannabis if you choose.

2.   Boil the water and pour it over the dry ingredients in the bowl. Cover and allow this to sit overnight or 6 - 8 hours.

3.   Put the mixture on the stove and heat on medium for 10 minutes. Using a masher, mash and pound the soapberry mixture to release the saponin liquid from the berries, which are now plump from water absorption. Set aside to cool. Use a strainer or cloth bag to strain the mixture, squeezing out as much liquid as possible, and set the leftovers aside.

4.   Prepare a muslin cloth or coffee filter to use in your strainer, and pour the liquid through it to remove

excess plant material. At this point you have a very concentrated soap liquid that is ready to be bottled. Add essential oils if you prefer. Two drops or more of any essential oil is best if you want to add fragrance to this gentle cleanser.

Keep this cleanser refrigerated when not in use. Don't panic if you forget it for a couple of days! It won't go bad that quickly, but it does require refrigeration to maintain freshness.

TIP* Take the leftover soapberry mixture and combine with a bowl or basin of warm water. Agitate, strain, and use this secondary strain right away to wash your hair or body!

The Perfect Conditioning Hair Oil

Not a soapberry recipe, but this is the perfect conditioning treatment to use after washing your hair with the soapberry shampoo. Never use bottled conditioner again!

TIP* You can also use this recipe as a scalp treatment for an irritated or itchy scalp by adding 1 tbsp or 15 ml of Cannabis Foundation Oil. This treatment should only be used on the scalp before washing hair and not after, as the cannabis oils are a bit too sticky to serve as a hair conditioner.

You will need:

2 tbsp or 30 ml of hemp seed oil

1/4 cup or 60 ml of sunflower oil

2 tbsp or 30 ml murumuru butter

2 drops of any cinnamon essential oil

2 drops of lemon or orange essential oil

1 drop of amber essential oil or paste (If amber resin or essential amber oil / paste is not available substitute with 1 drop each frankincense & myrrh essential oils.)

Preparation:

1.   Melt all of the oils together until warm and liquid, then add the essential oils as desired. Pour into a glass bottle or container. Shake well. This oil can be stored in cool dark place for up to 3 months.

Use a small amount to start and massage it into damp hair, starting with the ends of your hair and working up to the scalp. Comb the oil through and dry or style as usual.

Soapberries at Home

If you'd like an effective, healthy and environmentally friendly way to clean up and disinfect, soapberries are great!

Excellent for laundry, dishwashers, and as a general home cleanser, soapberries are anti-microbial and do a great job on dirt and odors, without exposing you or your family to any preservatives or petrochemicals!

For very greasy stains or cleaning jobs, you should use an orange-based degreaser before washing with soapberries.

Soapberry Thieves

Based on a very popular article from hempista.com about using essential oils as a disinfectant, and how modern hospitals are using the same "technology." This disinfectant is based on a recipe reputed to be from the Middle Ages, called 4 Thieves Vinegar.

Legend has it that the thieves were able to rob the dead during the black plague and not catch the disease by using vinegar that was steeped with certain herbs. At some point they were finally caught, and in a bargain made to spare their lives, they revealed the recipe that enabled their profitable exploits amongst the dead. The recipe that has been handed down throughout the centuries since then consists of essential oils known to be antimicrobial and antiviral, specifically: lavender, thyme, citrus and rosemary.

It's easy to recreate this healthy disinfectant using a few drops of essential oils, hot water and soapberries!

You will need:

Essential oils - lavender, thyme, lemon and rosemary

5 or more whole dried Sapindus Mukorossi soapberries, broken into two or more pieces.

Preparation:

Run scalding water in a bucket over the dried soap berries and add 2 drops of each essential oil. Agitate until sudsy. The soapberries may be removed later and used in another portion of disinfectant, so don't throw them out! They are usually good for 3 - 4 average size buckets of disinfecting cleaner.

In the Dishwasher or Hand Washing Dishes

Soapberries are great for soaking, washing dishes and the

dishwasher too. Add a few to your dish pan or to the utensil holder in your dishwasher.

Laundry

Throw 4 - 5 shelled soapberries in a muslin bag and toss in the washer. To whiten laundry, add oxygen "bleach." Treat stains before laundering by using a natural orange oil stain treatment.

Chapter 2: Lotions, Creams & Scrubs

Learn how to make cannabis topicals with both simple and luxurious ingredients!

Cannabis lotion, creams and scrubs are some of the best ways to enjoy the healing and beauty benefits of externally applied cannabis without any psychoactive effect.

All of the recipes are fully decarboxylated and rich in oleic acids, which is the key component in delivering cannabinoids externally in these recipes. All ingredients listed here are fully explained in Chapter 1 and can be sourced using the resources directory at the end of the book. In my personal experience, most ingredients are readily available locally.

The Secret of Ancients

Kaneh Bosem Anointing Oil for the Healing of the Nations

In 1936, as cannabis and hemp were about to become illegal for the first time in the United States, a Polish anthropologist who studied Judaic culture, Sula Benet, suggested that *kaneh bosem* - mentioned throughout the Bible - was not reed calamus as most scholars believe, but rather the fragrant cannabis-hemp "reed." This debate continues even today.

Then the LORD said to Moses, "Take the following fine spices: 500 shekels of liquid myrrh, half as much of fragrant cinnamon, 250 shekels of kaneh bosem, 500 shekels of cassia - all according to the sanctuary shekel – and a hind of olive oil. Make these into a sacred anointing oil"   Exodus 30: 22-33

Did the holy anointing oil prescribed by G-d for the priests in the Old Testament, and used generously to heal the sick by Jesus in the New Testament, contain cannabis? I don't know the answer to that question, but I suspect that it did.

The cannabis var. indica plant, a highly psychoactive and fragrant strain, is native to central Asia. Sula Benet's interpretation makes sense in light of the fragrance and other qualities described in the original texts. The fragrance profile of cannabis var. indica is unique in that its flowers have such a wide range of possible fragrances that are quite powerful, including fruits, spices, coffee, vanilla, lavender, citrus peels and more.

For me the proof lies in the effectiveness of the healing qualities of the formulation as written in the holy texts. Kaneh Bosem Healing Oil is my go-to oil when my joint pain levels are at their worst. There is a synergy between cannabis and the other essential oils in this preparation that is, in my opinion, unparalleled for pain relief.

The combination of herbs in this ancient recipe create a wellness formula that is very effective, yet simple enough to make at home.

The Herbs

Cassia and Cinnamon Bark Essential Oils - The kaneh bosem anointing oil recipe calls for two fragrant trees that produce what is commonly known today as cinnamon. Most cinnamon that is available on the grocery shelves is in fact cassia cinnamon, a cheaper variety.

True Ceylon cinnamon (Cinnamomum verum or Cinnamomum zeylanicum) is more rare and has a different fragrance from cassia, which is slightly more floral or sweet. Both of these cinnamon essential oils are used together in this recipe to create a warming and soothing sensation that increases circulation in painful joints.

Myrrh is an ancient tree resin from the Middle East that is used in fragrances, incense and mouthwash. It has anti-inflammatory and anti-microbial properties. It also has a very earthy scent that pairs well with cannabis. This recipe calls for myrrh essential oil in addition to cinnamon and cassia oils.

Olive Oil - The most common oil available in biblical times was also very high in oleic acid. And as we know, oleic acids are great for aiding in the absorption of cannabinoids from external preparations.

Kaneh bosem or cannabis *(It's no mistake that those names sound alike!)*. My favorite way to make Kaneh Bosem Healing Oil is with Rick Simpson Oil. It's the best pain relief recipe here! But for those that may not have access to the Simpson Oil, this recipe can be made with another Cannabis Foundation Oil from Chapter 1.

Kaneh Bosem Healing Oil

You will need:

1/2 cup or 120 ml of cold pressed, virgin olive oil

7 drops of myrrh essential oil

7 drops of common cassia cinnamon oil

5 drops of true Ceylon cinnamon essential oil (Cinnamomum verum or Cinnamomum zeylanicum)

1/2 cup or 120 ml Cannabis Foundation Oil made with olive oil (The Full-Extract Cannabis Oil or "Simpson Oil" recipe from Chapter 1 produces the best results.)

Preparation:

Thoroughly combine all ingredients and store in the refrigerator. This will partially solidify into a semi-soft ointment, and will still be easy to stir. Stir this ointment thoroughly before use. This healing oil may be used right from the jar, or you can prepare convenient lotion bars, or a fluffy refrigerated cold cream.

When this oil is used directly without further dilution in bars or lotions it is very concentrated with essential oils and cannabinoids. A small amount goes a long way and is even more effective when used with hot, moist towel wraps, or after a hot shower or bath.

Cannabis Lotion Bars

Lotion bars are easy to make and very portable! If this is your first time making lotions or creams, starting with lotion bars is quite satisfying and foolproof. The lotion bar recipes in this book are a lush treat and easy to make.

Lotion bars are best refrigerated, but because they don't contain water, they are shelf-stable for about 3 months.

Silicon muffin moulds work great for making lotion bars if you don't have any soap or candy moulds.

Simple Herbs Recovery Bar

This recipe uses warming herbs along with fats high in oleic acid to create a solid bar that's great to use on sore muscles or any time.

This bar contains a vegan floral wax from the tuberose flower. You may substitute with beeswax (not vegan) or another vegan wax, if you prefer.

Tuberose floral wax is a speciality wax that can be ordered online using the resource guide at the end of this book. It has a pleasant scent that is slightly medicinal and floral.

This recipe contains cayenne pepper and should not be used near the eyes or other mucus membranes.

Makes 3 - 4 bars.

You will need:

1/2 cup or 120 ml of mango seed butter

1/2 cup or 120 ml of tucuma or murumuru butter

1/4 cup or 60 ml of Cannabis Foundation Oil (Chapter 1)

3 tbsp or 45 ml of tuberose floral wax or beeswax

1 tsp or 2 grams of cayenne pepper powder

10 drops of ginger essential oil

10 drops of any cinnamon essential oil

Preparation:

1.   Melt the butters and wax together along with the cayenne pepper powder. After melting the butters and wax, add the cannabis oil and essential oils. Pour into moulds immediately.

2.   Allow to cool on the counter and then transfer to the refrigerator for a more solid bar that can easily be popped away from the mould.

Store wrapped in parchment paper in the refrigerator for up to 6 months. These bars are shelf stable for about 90 days.

Thai Stick Lemongrass Scrub Bar

Really awesome for scrubbing scaly irritated skin, this coarse lotion bar brings together the great qualities of the Thai Stick Lemongrass Lotion recipe in bar form, with coarse demerara sugar crystals for a great exfoliating treatment that's healing, soothing and sweet, just like the cannabis strain it's named after.

Makes 3 - 4 bars.

You will need:

1/2 cup or 120 ml of mango seed butter

1/2 cup or 120 ml of tucuma or murumuru butter

2 tbsp or 25 grams of coarse demerara sugar crystals

Leftover plant material from making Cannabis Foundation Oil (Chapter 1)

1 tbsp or 15 ml of tuberose floral wax or beeswax

15 drops lemongrass essential oil

Preparation:

1.   Melt the butter and wax together. Add the cannabis and lemongrass oil to the melted butter and wax.

2.   Add the sugar and stir briskly, then immediately pour into moulds and cool first on the counter and then in the refrigerator for a more solid bar. The bottom side of the bar will have a concentration of sugar crystals and cannabis herb when it hardens. Use this side for scrubbing.

Store these bars wrapped in baking parchment in the refrigerator for up to 6 months. These bars, like the other bar recipes, are stable at room temperature for about 3 months.

Cannabis Beauty Bar

Looking for a really lush and sensual beauty bar that smells divine? These cannabis beauty bars have a classic fragrance based on natural jasmine floral waxes and essential oils.

Makes 3 - 4 bars.

You will need:

1/2 cup or 120 ml of mango seed butter

1/2 cup or 120 ml of tucuma or murumuru butter

1/4 cup or 60 ml of Cannabis Foundation Oil (Chapter 1)

3 tbsp or 45 ml jasmine floral wax or beeswax

10 drops of amber or jasmine essential oil

2 drops of true Ceylon cinnamon essential oil (Cinnamomum verum or Cinnamomum zeylanicum)

Preparation:

1.   Melt the butters and wax together and add the cannabis oil and essential oils after the butters and wax have melted. Pour into moulds immediately.

2.   Allow to cool on the counter and then transfer to the refrigerator for a more solid bar that can easily be popped away from the mould.

Store wrapped in parchment paper in the refrigerator for up to 6 months. These bars are shelf stable for about 90 days.

Kaneh Bosem Lotion Bar

One of my favorite ways to enjoy the healing benefits of this ancient medicine is in a lotion bar. Because they are so portable, these bars are perfect for hikes and any strenuous exercise, to relieve pain during and after activities.

Makes 3 - 4 bars.

You will need:

1/4 cup or 60 ml of mango seed butter

1/2 cup or 120 ml of tucuma or murumuru butter

1/4 cup or 60 ml beeswax

1/2 cup or 120 ml Kaneh Bosem Healing Oil

5 drops of myrrh essential oil

5 drops of true Ceylon cinnamon essential oil (Cinnamomum verum or Cinnamomum zeylanicum)

5 drops of common cassia cinnamon oil

Preparation:

1.	Melt the butters and wax together and add the cannabis oil and essential oils after the butters and wax have melted. Pour into moulds immediately.

2.	Allow to cool on the counter and then transfer to the refrigerator for a more solid bar that can easily be popped away from the mould.

Store wrapped in parchment paper in the refrigerator for up to 6 months. These bars are shelf stable for about 90 days.

Paradise Tanning Lotion Bars

Cannabis has many known anti-cancer properties which makes it a great choice for sun-kissed skin.

There are two formulas to suit your tanning needs: The Tropical Paradise (humid tanning) and The Desert Paradise (dry tanning). Both formulas use exotic floral waxes and seed butters high in oleic acid along with cannabis to create paradise on your skin!

These tanning lotion bars are deeply moisturizing and are great after the sun too. Please note that these bars do not contain any SPF-rated sunscreen and are not intended to be used for that purpose.

The Tropical Paradise Tanning Lotion Bar

This bar incorporates tuberose floral wax, which gives it a golden color when used exclusively in a recipe with blonde keif or hashish. Ground cannabis flower will lend a green cast to this lotion bar.

Either way, the bar will apply a beautiful and sheer golden color to the skin due to the tuberose floral wax content.

Makes 3 - 4 bars.

You will need:

1 cup or 240 ml of cold pressed cocoa butter

1/4 cup or 60 ml of Cannabis Foundation Oil, made with sunflower oil for the best results (Chapter 1)

3 tbsp or 45 ml of tuberose floral wax or beeswax (Beeswax may be substituted in a pinch, but the tuberose floral wax is what gives this bar its unique color and scent.)

10 drops of ylang ylang essential oil

Preparation:

1.   Melt the cocoa butter and tuberose wax together. Add the cannabis oil and combine thoroughly with the ylang ylang essential oil.

2.   Pour into moulds and allow to cool on the counter, and then transfer to the refrigerator for a more solid bar that can easily be popped away from the mould.

Store wrapped in parchment paper in the refrigerator for up to 6 months. These bars are shelf stable for about 90 days.

The Desert Paradise Tanning Lotion Bar

Makes 3 - 4 small bars.

You will need:

1/2 cup or 120 ml of mango seed butter

1/2 cup or 120 ml of tucuma or murumuru butter

1/4 cup or 60 ml of Cannabis Foundation Oil (Chapter 1)

3 tbsp or 45 ml of jasmine floral wax or beeswax

5 drops jasmine essential oil

10 drops henna flower attar

2 drops amber essential oil or paste (A small piece of amber resin equivalent can be substituted.)

3 drops of lemon essential oil

Preparation:

1.   Melt the mango butter and jasmine wax together. Add the cannabis oil and combine thoroughly with the jasmine, henna and amber essential oils.

2.   Pour into moulds and allow to cool on the counter, and then transfer to the refrigerator for a more solid bar that can easily be popped away from the mould.

Store wrapped in parchment paper in the refrigerator for up to 6 months. These bars are shelf stable for about 90 days.

The Apothecary Cannabis Rose Recipes

Apothecary Rose, also known as Rose Gallica and Medieval Rose, is a small-medium ancient heirloom rose with a strong fragrance and color that varies from dark red to pink. This rose is a favorite for teas, herbal medicine and beauty. It's closely related to the Damascus rose and other varieties of rose that are used in commercial oil and hydrosol production.

These cannabis rose recipes are based on the Apothecary Rose, which is known for its skin emollient and wrinkle minimizing properties. These recipes rely on essential rose oils, fats, waxes and hydrosols for their unique properties and fragrance.

When working with cannabis oils, it's important to round out the sharp herbal scent of cannabis with other fragrances so the fragrances are not overpowered by the scent of the cannabis. Cannabis scents should play nicely with all the other scents, and the oils shouldn't leave you smelling like your favorite cannabis dispensary!

The Apothecary Cannabis Rose recipes do just that. With the addition of true Ceylon cinnamon oil, the sharper notes of the cannabis flower take a step back to reveal a gorgeous rose fragrance that's natural and not overpowering. This cinnamon has a fruity almost floral quality that sets it apart from the more common cassia variety of cinnamon, and plays extraordinarily well with the other flowers in these recipes.

Apothecary Cannabis Rose Lotion Bar

These bars have an amazing ability to maintain their fragrance even when they are left in the open air, as I have done so many times. Nevertheless, if you want to maintain the best fragrance, store these in wrapped parchment baking paper or bags.

Makes 3 - 4 small bars.

You will need:

1/2 cup or 120 ml of mango seed butter

1/2 cup or 120 ml tucuma or murumuru butter

1/4 cup or 60 ml of Cannabis Foundation Oil (Chapter 1)

3 tbsp or 45 ml rose floral wax or beeswax

5 drops true Ceylon cinnamon essential oil (Cinnamomum verum or Cinnamomum zeylanicum)

10 drops rose or geranium rose essential oil

Preparation:

1.   Melt the butters and wax together and add the cannabis oil and essential oils after the butters and wax have melted. Pour into moulds immediately.

2.   Allow to cool on the counter, and then transfer to the refrigerator for a more solid bar that can easily be popped away from the mould.

Store wrapped in parchment paper in the refrigerator for up to 6 months. These bars are shelf stable for about 90 days.

Apothecary Cannabis Rose Ancient Salt Scrub Bar

This lively exfoliating scrub will take your tired and sallow skin from sad to fabulous! This scrub is fantastic to use before taking one of the cannabis baths in Chapter 3.

Makes 3 - 4 small bars.

You will need:

1/2 cup or 120 ml of mango seed butter

1/2 cup or 120 ml tucuma or murumuru butter

1 tbsp or 15 ml rose floral wax or beeswax

Leftover ground flower material from making the Cannabis Foundation Oil (Chapter 1)

2 drops of true Ceylon cinnamon essential oil (Cinnamomum verum or Cinnamomum zeylanicum)

5 drops rose or geranium rose essential oil

5 drops essential lemon oil

1/4 cup or 60 grams ancient sea salt or Himalayan salt, fine to semi-coarse grind

Preparation:

1.   Gently melt the butters and rose wax together. Add the cannabis, salt and essential oils as the last step before pouring into moulds.

2.   Cool on the counter until almost hard, and then place in the refrigerator until they are hard enough to remove from the moulds. The salt and cannabis herbs will collect on the bottom of the bars while cooling to create a perfect scrub side!

Store unused bars in the refrigerator up to 6 months. This bar will keep well in normal room temperatures for about 90 days.

Chocolate & Roses Lip Balm

Meet your new favorite lip balm! Valentine's Day is every day when you wear this tasty and very kissable cannabis lip balm. This recipe makes a solid balm that can be poured into a lip balm dispenser or into a small cosmetic lip gloss pot.

You will need:

2 tbsp or 30 ml of cold-pressed and raw cacao butter

2 tbsp or 30 ml of Cannabis Foundation Oil – made with sunflower oil (Chapter 1)

1 tbsp or 15 ml of rose floral wax (Don't substitute this time, this rose floral wax gives this balm its flavor and moisture.)

1 drop of true Ceylon cinnamon essential oil (Cinnamomum verum or Cinnamomum zeylanicum)

Preparation:

Melt the butter and wax. Add the cannabis oil and cinnamon oil, stir and then pour into a container. Finish by letting the preparation set in the refrigerator.

This lip balm has a shelf life of roughly 2 months if carried in your purse or pocket frequently. Otherwise, stored in a cool, dark place it should last for up to 3 months.

Making Creams and Lotions

Creams and lotions contain enough water that when exposed to normal shelf storage conditions they will become hotbeds of microbial activity if they do not have preservatives. All off-the-shelf commercial cream and lotion products, organic or not, contain preservatives.

As explained in Chapter 1, preservatives may be avoided by creating small batches, keeping the product in refrigeration, and using it within 30 days. This small batch philosophy applies to all of the lotion recipes made with high quality food-grade ingredients.

Proper emulsification is another requirement for successful batches of lotions and creams, which guarantees that the moisturizing elements of the lotions and creams will not separate from the oils. There are two critical principles for proper emulsification:

1.   All ingredients must be at the same temperature before mixing, typically around 140 F or 60 C.

2.   An emulsifying agent must be present. In these recipes, sunflower lecithin and sometimes wax are the emulsifiers of choice.

By bringing all ingredients to the same temperature in a liquid state, and using the emulsifying agents, these ingredients become luxurious cannabis lotions and creams!

Simple (But Powerful) Cannabis Lotion

The easiest way to make cannabis lotion is to use the concentrated Cannabis Foundation Oil from Chapter 1 and just 3 other ingredients. Try it!

You will need:

1/4 cup or 60 ml of Cannabis Foundation Oil (Chapter 1)

1/2 tsp or 2 grams of sunflower lecithin

1 cup of preservative-free aloe vera juice

1 tsp or 5 ml lemon juice

Any essential oils you prefer

Preparation:

1.   Gently heat the cannabis oil and melt the sunflower lecithin in the oil until dissolved. At the same time, warm the aloe vera juice and lemon juice to the same temperature as the oil, 140 F or 60 C.

2.   Pour the hot oil in a bowl and begin mixing with a whisk or hand mixer while slowly pouring in the hot aloe vera juice. Mix and add essential oils until creamy. This will make a very milky lotion. Store in the refrigerator for up to 30 days.

Apothecary Cannabis Rose Cold Cream

This is a thick moisturizing cold cream reminiscent of the rose cold creams of the 1950's. This cold cream should remain refrigerated, which not only extends its freshness, but also makes it extremely refreshing when applied to the skin after a hot shower or spa.

You will need:

1/2 cup or 120 ml of mango seed butter

1/2 cup or 120 ml of Cannabis Foundation Oil – made with sunflower oil for best results (Chapter 1)

1 tbsp or 15 ml of rose floral wax or beeswax

1 tsp or 5 grams of sunflower lecithin

1/4 cup or 60 ml distilled rose water

1/4 cup or 60 ml of aloe vera gel, scraped from the leaf

5 drops true Ceylon cinnamon essential oil (Cinnamomum verum or Cinnamomum zeylanicum)

10 drops essential rose or rose geranium oil

1 tsp or 5 ml lemon juice

Preparation:

1.   Combine rose water, lemon juice and the aloe vera gel until smooth in the blender. Pour into a pan and heat to about 140 F or 60 C.

2.   Melt the wax, mango seed butter, sunflower lecithin and cannabis oil in a separate pan on the stove. Heat this mixture to about 140 F or 60 C.

3.   Pour the hot oil and wax mixture into a mixing bowl, and mix with a hand mixer or stand mixer for the best results. Slowly add the hot rose water combination to the oils while mixing on high. Add all of the essential oils while mixing until creamy and fluffy.

TIP* Refrigerate and then whip again on high for an extra-fluffy cream. The cream will stiffen up a bit as it cools in the refrigerator. Store this cream in the refrigerator and use within 30 days.

Apothecary Cannabis Rose Milk

A milky and quick absorbing lotion that will leave the slightest scent of roses, Apothecary Cannabis Rose Milk makes a great everyday moisturizer for the face or hands.

You will need:

2 tbsp or 30 ml mango seed butter

1/4 cup or 60 ml of Cannabis Foundation Oil – made with sunflower oil for best results (Chapter 1)

1/2 tsp or 2 grams of sunflower lecithin

1/2 cup or 120 ml distilled rose water

1/4 cup or 60 ml of aloe vera gel, scraped from the leaf

2 drops true Ceylon cinnamon essential oil (Cinnamomum verum or Cinnamomum zeylanicum)

3 drops essential rose or rose geranium oil

1 tsp or 5 ml lemon juice

Preparation:

1.   In a blender, combine rose water, lemon juice and the aloe vera gel for a few seconds until thoroughly smooth. Pour into a pan on the stove, and heat to about 140 F or 60 C.

2.   Melt the wax, mango seed butter, sunflower lecithin and cannabis oil in a separate pan on the stove. Heat this mixture to about 140 F or 60 C.

3.   Pour the hot oil and wax mixture into a mixing bowl, and mix with a hand mixer or stand mixer for the best results. Slowly add the hot rose water combination to the oils while mixing on high. Add all of the essential oils while mixing until creamy and smooth.

Store this lotion in the refrigerator and use within 30 days.

Recovery Pain Cream

This is a thick medicated cream that's even better when used with a moist, hot towel wrap.

This cream contains three intensive anti-inflammatory herbs: ginger, turmeric and cannabis. It's really great for sports injuries and sore muscles too. I love the muscle healing warmth of this cream after any workout or exercise session. This recovery cream will add a temporary golden glow to the skin due to the presence of turmeric.

You will need:

1/4 cup or 60 ml of mango seed butter

1/2 cup or 120 ml of Cannabis Foundation Oil (Chapter 1)

1/4 cup or 60 ml of aloe vera gel, scraped from the leaf

1/4 cup or 60 ml of orange flower water

1 tsp or 5 grams of sunflower lecithin

1 tbsp or 5 grams of powdered turmeric

10 drops essential ginger oil

10 drops of any cinnamon oil

1 tsp or 5 ml lemon juice

Preparation:

1.   In a blender, combine orange flower water, lemon juice, turmeric powder and the aloe vera gel for a few seconds until thoroughly smooth. Pour into a pan on the stove, and heat to about 140 F or 60 C.

2.   Melt the mango seed butter, sunflower lecithin and cannabis oil in a separate pan on the stove. Heat this mixture to about 140 F or 60 C.

3.   Pour the hot oil and butter mixture into a mixing bowl, and mix with a hand mixer or stand mixer for the best results. Slowly add the hot orange flower water and aloe vera combination to the oils while mixing on high. Add

all of the essential oils while mixing until creamy and smooth.

TIP* Refrigerate and then whip again on high for an extra-fluffy cream.

The cream will stiffen up a bit as it cools in the refrigerator. Store this cream in the refrigerator and use within 30 days.

Thai Stick Lemongrass Lotion

Reminiscent of the earlier years of the drug war when the legendary Thai strains or "Thai Sticks" were a hot commodity, if you could get them! This lotion was made for a great sativa strain, so use the Cannabis Foundation Oil from Chapter 1 that has been made with dried and ground Thai strains of cannabis flowers.

This recipe uses both fresh lemongrass stalks and fresh aloe vera leaves. The advantage of this is that the lotion is not only a great moisturizer, but also a great bug repellent that's good for your skin!

You will need:

2 tbsp or 30 ml mango seed butter

1/4 cup or 60 ml of Cannabis Foundation Oil (Chapter 1)

1/2 cup or 120 ml aloe vera gel, scraped from the leaf

1/2 cup or 120 ml distilled water or spring water

3 stalks of fresh lemongrass with the green cut away

1/2 tsp or 2 grams of sunflower lecithin

10 drops of lemongrass essential oil

1 tsp or 5 ml lemon juice

Preparation:

1.   Cut up the lemongrass stalks and scrape the gel from the fresh aloe vera leaves. Blend the water and lemongrass stalks in a blender until almost smooth. Filter all of the solids from the liquid. Put the liquid back in the blender with the aloe vera gel and lemon juice, and blend until smooth. Heat this liquid to 140 F or 60 C on the stove.

2.   Melt the wax, sunflower lecithin, mango seed butter and cannabis oil in a separate pan. Heat this mixture to 140 F or 60 C.

3.   Pour the hot oil mixture into a mixing bowl, and mix with a hand mixer or stand mixer for the best results. Slowly add the hot aloe vera, lemon juice and lemongrass combination to the oils while mixing on high. Add all of the essential oils while mixing until creamy and smooth.

Store this lotion in the refrigerator and use within 30 days.

Kaneh Bosem Desert Caravan Cold Cream

Another simple recipe that can be made with the basic Kaneh Bosem Healing Oil recipe.

You will need:

1/2 cup or 120 ml of mango seed butter

1/2 cup or 120 ml Kaneh Bosem Healing Oil

1/4 cup or 60 ml of aloe vera gel, scraped from the leaf

1/4 cup or 60 ml of distilled orange flower water

1 tsp or 5 grams of sunflower lecithin

2 drops of any cinnamon essential oil

5 drops of essential orange or lemon oil

1 tsp or 5 ml lemon juice

Preparation:

1.   In the blender combine the lemon juice, orange flower water and aloe vera until smooth. Heat this mixture in a pan on the stove to 140 F or 60 C. Melt the sunflower lecithin, butter and cannabis oil in a pan on the stove at 140 F or 60 C.

2.   Pour the hot oil mixture into a mixing bowl, and mix with a hand mixer or stand mixer for the best results. Slowly add the hot aloe vera and orange flower water combination to the oils while mixing on high. Add all of the essential oils while mixing until creamy and smooth.

Store this lotion in the refrigerator and use within 30 days.

Chapter 3: Getting High on Bath Salts

(No, really!)

There. I knew that would get your attention! But, I'm not talking about THOSE bath salts. Cannabis won't turn you into a zombie. I promise!

These cannabis bath salts are soothing, anti-inflammatory, non-drying, and luscious on the skin. And if you are seeking pain relief from a number of conditions like arthritis, chronic headaches, cramps or nerve pain, these baths will leave you refreshed and feeling fantastic.

It's hard to smile when you are in pain. A smile is guaranteed with every one of these baths.

Caveat: These bath preparations do have the potential to relax your muscles and induce euphoria depending on the concentration of cannabinoids used and the length of time you spend in the bath. Please avoid driving or operating heavy machinery after bathing. Allow 3 - 8 hours depending on the concentration of cannabinoids you have absorbed. These baths may also be adjusted so they have no psychoactive effect at all, but still provide benefits that are similar to lotions.

You can prepare the bath salts in any cannabinoid concentration you prefer, there is no upward limit. However, you may need to adjust other ingredients to ensure the cannabis oils have been fully emulsified. More than the suggested amount can be wasteful. The effects of this bath have more to do with soaking time (exposure) than deploying super-concentrations of cannabinoids.

You should spend as much time soaking in this bath as you feel is necessary. Based on the experience of those that have tried this bath, the consensus is that you will begin to feel the benefits of this bath in 15 minutes, with typical soak times being between 30 - 60 minutes for maximum benefit.

The Bath Salts Story

I am frequently asked how I came up with these bath salt recipes! Like a lot of other interesting inventions, it was somewhat by accident.

I have used many bath salts from the legal dispensaries and I have also attempted to make my own using standard bath bomb and salt techniques. The problem with these methods is that the cannabis oils either float on top of the water for a lovely "ring around the tub," or they end up encapsulated in some form of starch, neither of which creates a fully emulsified bath that *really* penetrates into your tissues.

Having some previous knowledge of the power of saponins as a surfactant that emulsifies the oils and keeps them emulsified, in addition to being a powerful agent to increase absorption of essential oils transdermally, I started experimenting with traditional folk herbal saponins like soapberries. I made my first soapberry cannabis bath base, mixed it up with salt, and was very excited to try the results.

I was initially aiming for non-psychoactive pain relief like the lotion recipes. I soaked in the tub for about an hour before I was scheduled to drive my car to an appointment. Well, that was a wash, literally! About 15 minutes after getting out of that powerful bath, I was too euphoric to drive!

Now, I'm more careful, of course. :)

The Key Features of the Bath Salts Recipe:

1.   Emulsion and even distribution of oils in the formula.

Emulsion is the process of combining oils and water by using a third and/or fourth ingredient, in this case, surfactants (Sapindus Mukorossi), mucilage (Aloe Vera) and sunflower lecithin to firm up the emulsion. The oils stay emulsified and active when added to bathwater. No ring around the tub or wasted oils that float on the surface.

2.   Fully decarboxylated cannabis oils and extracts.

Decarboxylation happens when cannabinoids are heated and shed a carbon atom. All of the recipes include this important step to ensure that the cannabinoids are fully bioactive.

3.   A low-foaming formula that works well with salt crystals.

These baths can be used in jetted tubs or soaking tubs. They are high in saponins, which come from the soapberries, and will not foam heavily in a jetted tub. You may get some light foaming which will dissipate fairly quickly.

Making cannabis bath salts is a two-step process:

1.   Making the concentrated cannabis bath base.

2.   Adding the concentrated cannabis bath base to a salt and aloe vera mixture and finishing with desired essential oils and/or teas.

Making the Cannabis Bath Base

We will start with fresh, authentic, dried, de-seeded Sapindus Mukorossi berries. In Chapter 1, I talk about what these berries are and where you can obtain them. They are part of the traditional Ayurvedic pharmacopoeia, and have been used for thousands of years for skin and hair health.

Soapberries are unique in the way their saponins interact with cannabinoids in water. This makes them perfect for bath formulations. They are noted for their anti-inflammatory and anti-microbial properties, which nicely complements the cannabis herb when used together.

Sapindus Mukorossi has the two most important qualities necessary to create a superior bath formula for our purposes: it's low-foaming and high in saponins.

Do not substitute other surfactants or soap products.

Do not use any pre-prepared soapberry product.

Use only the raw product and prepare the soapberries according to this recipe for the best results.

Sapindus Mukorossi has a distinctive, pleasant "cooked pineapple" or "apple cider vinegar" fragrance when it's cooked by itself. You may be able to detect the fragrance of cannabis before the scent of the soapberries in a full bath. In these recipes, I prepare the bath base with lemon peel and lavender to round out the fragrance of the soapberries and cannabis.

This enhances the aromatherapy experience of each of the custom bath recipes that follow the basic recipes. The base prepared this way can also be used alone in a bath with no essential oils or spices for a virtually fragrance-free bath.

My bath recipes include mostly easy-to-source ingredients, detailed in Chapter 1. I do include some exotic ingredients, like flower attars, which may be sourced from the resource guide at the end of this book or online. The resource guide contains the sources I trust for authentic and fresh ingredients which work well in my test kitchen when making each of these recipes.

This base recipe is not shelf-stable and requires refrigeration. Failure to refrigerate can result in microbial contamination. This is a small batch recipe that will make 3 - 5 baths depending on your preferences.

The bath base has a shelf life of about 1 - 2 weeks in the refrigerator. To avoid microbial contamination, any bath salts you make should be refrigerated and used within 1 - 2 weeks for the best results.

Salt inhibits many bad organisms, but not all. Without preservatives, this is a perishable product. Alternatively, you may freeze the baths or bath base portions for storage up to 6 months.

TIP* Roughly speaking, for each bath, if using near the high end of the suggested cannabis amounts, the bath will contain about a hashish-gram or more worth of cannabinoids.

I typically make 5 bath portions at a time, and each one will contain the cannabinoid equivalent of a gram of hashish. The suggested amounts in this recipe will vary depending on your preferences. This bath recipe can be as intensive or as gentle as you prefer.

My typical routine is to immerse my entire body, head and all! The soapberry formulation makes the bath a great cleanser for hair and body. Rinse in the shower briefly after taking a bath, if you prefer.

The Basic Cannabis Bath Base Recipe Using Dried and Finely Ground Cannabis Trim, Flowers, Hashish, or Keif

Makes 3 or more bath base portions.

TIP* Splitting this bath base into 5 portions, or even more if you have a low tolerance or have not used cannabis before (thereby using smaller concentrations of cannabinoids) will have the relieving and non-psychoactive effect of most cannabis lotions. 3 or less portions will intensify effects and may be psychoactive. Please plan your activities accordingly. Longer soak times intensify the effects of any portion size you choose.

You will need:

50 whole, de-seeded Sapindus Mukorossi berries (soapberry, aritha) split in half (If you are creating a bath base that is at the higher end of cannabinoid concentration, use more soapberries for better emulsification.)

1 quart or 1 litre of water

Lemon peels from one lemon

2 tbsp or 30 ml of aloe vera gel, scraped from the leaf

1 tbsp or 3 grams of dried lavender flowers or a few fresh sprigs of fresh lavender flowers

3 - 14 grams of potent, dried and finely ground cannabis flowers

OR

2 - 8 grams of hashish or keif

OR

10 - 28 grams cannabis trim, ground

1 tbsp or 15 ml olive or sunflower oil, or a little more if necessary. The addition of this oil should be just enough to fully saturate the plant or to dissolve the concentrate material.

1/4 tsp or 1 gram of sunflower lecithin

Preparation:

1.   Melt the sunflower lecithin in the oil. Pour this oil over the cannabis and allow it to marinate while you prepare the soapberries.

2.   Rinse the dried berries in warm water once, quickly, and drain. Add the soapberries, lemon peels and lavender to a bowl.

3.   Bring the water to a boil on the stove, and add to the ingredients in the bowl. Allow this to sit on the counter overnight or 6 - 8 hours to extract the saponins and other essential ingredients from the herbs.

4.   After this extraction, put the soapberry mixture on the stove and add the marinated cannabis and aloe vera gel which has been scraped from the fresh leaf. Cook this mixture while frequently mashing down and stirring until it reduces to about half as much liquid or less on medium heat. This will take about 15 - 30 minutes. The plant material should be mushy and pulpy at the end of this process.

5.   Remove and allow to cool to a warm-to-the-touch temperature. Using a strainer or cloth bag, extract as much juice as possible from the mixture in a bowl. This is your first and strongest bath base mixture. Set aside but do not refrigerate yet.

You should have about 1 - 2 cups or 240 - 480 ml of thick, gravy-like liquid.

The berries and cannabis flower material that is left over will be set aside for a second extraction which is used in the poultice, wrap, foot and hand soak recipes.

Additionally, you may use the second or even third extractions for a full bath as well. Extract again using a quart or pint of boiling water, cool, and strain as before. Use this as a base for any of the bath recipes.

The Basic Cannabis Bath Base Recipe Using Full-extract Decarboxylated Cannabis Oil ("Simpson Oil")

Makes 3 or more bath base portions.

Full-extract cannabis oil is a fully decarboxylated cannabis oil that normally uses alcohol in the extraction process, which is then boiled off to create a thick and concentrated tar-like oil. I explain more about the origins and popularity of this oil in Chapter 1.

If you live in a location with legal cannabis dispensaries there is a good chance that you will be able to purchase this oil or have a caregiver make it for you.

This recipe is different than the basic bath base with raw cannabis because we do not need to take the oil through the long boiling process. The oil is thinned with olive or sunflower oil and added right before the soapberries have boiled down to a thick liquid.

TIP* Splitting this bath base into 5 portions, or even more if you have a low tolerance or have not used cannabis before (thereby using smaller concentrations of cannabinoids) will have the relieving and non-psychoactive effect of most cannabis lotions. 3 or less portions will intensify effects and may be psychoactive. Please plan your activities accordingly. Longer soak times intensify the effects of any portion size you choose.

You will need:

50 whole, de-seeded Sapindus Mukorossi berries (soapberry, aritha) split in half (If you are creating a bath base that is at the higher end of cannabinoid concentration, use more soapberries for better emulsification.)

1 quart or 1 litre of water

Lemon peels from one lemon

2 tbsp or 30 ml of aloe vera gel, scraped from the leaf

1 tbsp or 1 gram of dried lavender flowers or a few fresh sprigs of fresh lavender flowers

3 - 7 grams of full-extract cannabis oil ("Simpson Oil")

1 tbsp or 15 ml olive or sunflower oil, or a little more if necessary. The addition of this oil should be just enough to dilute the full-extract cannabis oil well enough to make it a bit thinner.

1/4 tsp or 1 gram of sunflower lecithin

Preparation:

1.   Melt the sunflower lecithin in the oil. Prepare the full-extract cannabis oil by dissolving in the olive or sunflower oil. Cover and set aside.

2.   Rinse the dried berries in warm water once, quickly. Add the soapberries, lemon peels and lavender to a bowl.

3.   Bring the water to a boil and add to the ingredients in the bowl. Allow this to sit on the counter overnight or 6 - 8 hours to extract the saponins and other essential ingredients from the herbs.

4.   After this extraction, put the soapberry mixture on the stove and cook on medium heat while frequently mashing down and stirring until it reduces to about half as much liquid or less, and becomes very pulpy. This will take about 15 - 30 minutes.

5.   Add the aloe vera gel that has been scraped from the leaf and the cannabis oil to the mixture on the stove, mash and cook for about 5 more minutes on low heat until the oil emulsifies into the thick liquid. Remove and allow to cool to a warm-to-the-touch temperature.

6.   Using a strainer or cloth bag, extract as much juice as possible from the mixture in a bowl. This is your first and strongest bath base mixture. Set aside, but do not refrigerate yet.

You should have about 1 - 2 cups or 240 - 480 ml of thick liquid.

As with the raw cannabis bath base, the leftover pulp from making this bath base can be used again in soaks, poultices, and even an additional extraction for a full bath.

The Bath Salt Recipes

You will want to make your bath salts as soon as your bath base has been strained and set aside. You will be adding essential oils and herbs at this point, and the bath base is best to work with when it is still slightly warm.

The Basic Bath Salt Recipe

The bath salt recipes that follow are all variations on this basic recipe.

Makes 1 bath.

You will need:

1 - 2 cups or 250 - 500 grams of coarse Himalayan pink salt, ancient salt, or sea salt for large soaking or jetted tubs

OR

1/2 cup - 1 cup or 125 - 250 grams of coarse Himalayan pink salt, ancient salt, or sea salt, for average size tubs

2 tbsp or 30 ml of aloe vera gel, scraped from the leaf

1 portion of the Cannabis Bath Base

Assorted essential oils, if desired

Preparation:

1.   Using a large mortar and pestle or large glass mixing bowl, pour in all of the salt.

2.   Scrape the gel from the aloe leaf and mash the aloe vera gel into the salt until dissolved. Add 1 portion of the cannabis bath base.

3.   Add drops of the essential oils of your choice to the salt bath and gently fold into the mixture.

That's it! Refrigerate for up to 2 weeks, freeze for up to 6 months, or use immediately.

If you would like to use spice or herbal teas like I do in the recipes that follow, brew these in a separate pan and add after boiling with medium heat, reducing the liquid to about 1/4 cup or 60 ml.

It's also important to note that the final result in your tub will have a different fragrance than the final concentrated bath salt portion. The scents of the soapberry, lemon peels, and lavender dissipate to reveal the fragrance of the essential oils and spices that have been added. As mentioned before, if your preference is a virtually fragrance free bath, use this basic bath salt recipe with no additional essential oils or spices.

TIP* To preserve the integrity of the essential oils in these bath recipes you'll need to put these baths in bottles or jars and refrigerate as soon as possible. Keep them tightly sealed.

The Moonshine Bath

My grandmother used to make a cake called Moonshine Cake. It didn't actually have any alcohol in it, but it hails from the era of 1930's prohibition. It's a decadent and delicately scented white cake. She passed down her tattered recipe card to me many years ago, and that's the inspiration for this bath recipe. It's totally decadent, just like the cake. Celebrate the end of cannabis prohibition today with this Moonshine Bath!

Speaking of which: if you're experiencing PMS what could be better than a big slice of decadent white cake with no calories? A delicious sugar high without the guilt!

The recipe uses lush amber paste and essential oils, in particular jasmine and amber. These are amongst the most luxurious fragrances available. You may substitute with another form of jasmine fragrance, but for the best results, you should use a jasmine essential oil.

Makes 1 bath.

You will need:

1 - 2 cups or 250 - 500 grams of coarse Himalayan pink salt, ancient salt, or sea salt for large soaking or jetted tubs

OR

1/2 cup - 1 cup or 125 - 250 grams of coarse Himalayan pink salt, ancient salt, or sea salt, for average size tubs

2 tbsp or 30 ml of aloe vera gel, scraped from the leaf

1 portion of the Cannabis Bath Base

3 drops of jasmine essential oil

3 drops of ylang ylang essential oil

1 drop of essential amber oil or resin paste (May substitute with 2 drops of frankincense.)

1 vanilla bean, scraped of seeds (Set aside the seed pulp and scraped bean separately.)

1 thumb of fresh ginger, chopped

1 bag or 2 grams of white tea

2 cups or 480 ml of water

Preparation:

1.   Using a large mortar and pestle or large glass mixing bowl, pour in all of the salt. Scrape the gel from the aloe leaf and mash the aloe vera gel into the salt until dissolved.

2.   In a pan on the stove, add the ginger, white tea, scraped vanilla bean, water, and boil using medium heat until there is only about 1/4 cup (60 ml) of concentrated liquid. Cool and strain.

3.   Add the bath base portion and the cooled spice & tea liquid to the salt while stirring.

4.   Add the essential oils and vanilla seed pulp as the last step and fold in gently.

Your finished bath salt will be wet to semi-liquid. Use immediately or store in the refrigerator. Seal this in a tight container in the refrigerator for up to 2 weeks or in the freezer for 6 months.

The Recovery Bath

This is a bath salt that I have personally employed against the evil pain of autoimmune disease. This bath is not for the faint of heart.

This bath also contains raw turmeric root in quantities which may stain your skin a very slight golden color. If you have a tan or darker skin, this will make you glow! But if you have lighter skin, you may notice a slight golden color. It doesn't last long but it will be present.

Turmeric is an essential part of this bath due to its anti-inflammatory properties. You may omit this ingredient but the results may vary because this is a key ingredient in this bath.

This bath is great for all kinds of recovery situations, including sports injury recovery.

Makes 1 bath.

You will need:

1 - 2 cups or 250 - 500 grams of coarse Himalayan pink salt, ancient salt, or sea salt for large soaking or jetted tubs

OR

1/2 cup - 1 cup or 125 - 250 grams of coarse Himalayan pink salt, ancient salt, or sea salt, for average size tubs

2 tbsp or 30 ml of aloe vera gel, scraped from the leaf

1 portion of the Cannabis Bath Base

5 drops of ginger essential oil

2 drops of lavender essential oil

3 drops of rosemary essential oil

2 drops of peppermint oil

3 drops of any cinnamon oil

1/4 cup or 60 grams of fresh grated turmeric root or 1 tbsp or 5 grams of turmeric powder

1 cup or 240 ml water

Preparation:

1.   Using a large mortar and pestle or large glass mixing bowl, pour in all of the salt. Scrape the gel from the aloe leaf and mash the aloe vera gel into the salt until dissolved.

2.   In a pan on the stove, add the turmeric and water and boil until there is about 1/4 cup (60 ml) of concentrated liquid. Allow to cool, and strain if necessary.

3.   Add the cannabis bath base and turmeric tea to the salt while stirring.

4.   Add the essential oils as the last step and fold in gently.

Your finished bath salt will be wet to semi-liquid. Use immediately or store in the refrigerator. Seal this in a tight container in the refrigerator for up to 2 weeks or in the freezer for 6 months.

Sultana's Bath

Inspired by the hammam traditions of the Middle East and Sufi poetry, Sultana's Bath is the perfect romance and relaxation bath.

This bath uses rose essential oil or "attar of rose," henna flower attar, amber and spices for an intoxicating scent that is like an oasis of beauty and love.

The earthy scent of the henna flower is included in this formula for warmth and grounding. Henna is renown in the desert climates for perfumery, sunscreen, skin health and beauty. You can find out how to acquire this exotic ingredient for Sultana's Bath and some of the other recipes in the resource directory at the end of this book.

Makes 1 bath.

You will need:

1 - 2 cups or 250 - 500 grams of coarse Himalayan pink salt, ancient salt, or sea salt for large soaking or jetted tubs

OR

1/2 cup - 1 cup or 125 - 250 grams of coarse Himalayan pink salt, ancient salt, or sea salt, for average size tubs

2 tbsp or 30 ml of aloe vera gel, scraped from the leaf

1 portion of the Cannabis Bath Base

3 drops of rose or geranium rose essential oil

3 drops henna flower attar

2 drops of amber essential oil or paste (If amber resin or essential amber oil / paste is not available substitute with 2 drops each frankincense & myrrh essential oils.)

1 cinnamon stick

5 cardamom pods, broken

3 clove buds

Dried blood orange peels from 1 orange or regular orange peels

10 threads of saffron

2 cups or 480 ml of water

Preparation:

1.   Using a large mortar and pestle or large glass mixing bowl, pour in all of the salt. Scrape the gel from the aloe leaf and mash the aloe vera gel into the salt until dissolved.

2.   In a pan on the stove, add all of the spices, water, and boil using medium heat until there is only about 1/4 cup (60 ml) of concentrated liquid. Cool and strain.

3.   Add the cannabis bath base and spice liquid to the salt and stir.

4.   Add the essential oils as the last step and fold in gently.

Your finished bath salt will be wet to semi-liquid. Use immediately or store in the refrigerator. Seal this in a tight container in the refrigerator for up to 2 weeks or in the freezer for 6 months.

Shiva's Bath

A spicy, citrusy and slightly floral bath inspired by the Hindu deity that also loves the sacred cannabis herb. This bath has a strong lingham vibration for the warrior, or the wounded. Perfect for man or woman.

Makes 1 bath.

You will need:

1 - 2 cups or 250 - 500 grams of coarse Himalayan pink salt, ancient salt, or sea salt for large soaking or jetted tubs

OR

1/2 cup - 1 cup or 125 - 250 grams of coarse Himalayan pink salt, ancient salt, or sea salt, for average size tubs

2 tbsp or 30 ml of aloe vera gel, scraped from the leaf

1 portion of the Cannabis Bath Base

2 drops of jasmine essential oil

5 drops of lemon essential oil

1 drop of amber essential oil or paste (If amber resin or essential amber oil / paste is not available substitute with 1 drop each frankincense & myrrh essential oils.)

2 drops of patchouli essential oil

1 cup of dried blood orange peels or regular orange peels

2 cinnamon sticks

1 star of anise

1 cardamom pod, cracked

1 thumb of fresh ginger, chopped or 1 tablespoon of ginger powder

1 tbsp (15 grams) or 2 bags of black tea

2 cups or 480 ml of water

Preparation:

1.   Using a large mortar and pestle or large glass mixing bowl, pour in all of the salt. Scrape the gel from the aloe leaf and mash the aloe vera gel into the salt until dissolved.

2.   In a pan on the stove, add all of the spices, water, and boil using medium heat until there is only about 1/4 cup (60 ml) of concentrated liquid. Cool and strain.

3.   Add the cannabis bath base and spice liquid to the salt and stir.

4.   Add the essential oils as the last step and fold in gently.

Your finished bath salt will be wet to semi-liquid. Use immediately or store in the refrigerator. Seal this in a tight container in the refrigerator for up to 2 weeks or in the freezer for 6 months.

Cannabis Soaks

That bowl of mush leftover from making cannabis bath base is now ready to be used to make these fabulous soaks!

After you extract most of the liquid from the plant material for your bath base portions, you will want to do one more extraction to release all of the plant saponins, fragrances and nutrients along with the remaining cannabinoids.

This extraction is perfect for foot spas and soaks and for my signature hand plunge technique. You may also extract one portion only from the leftover maceration and use this in a full bath with salt.

Additionally, in Chapter 4 there are more recipes for poultices and wraps that use this second extraction of the bath base.

Cannabis Soak Base

This extraction makes 3 portions.

Preparation:

1.   Add all leftover plant material, including any tea material to one pot with 1 quart or 1 litre of boiling water.

2.   Agitate and allow to cool for 2 - 3 hours. Strain.

3.   Split into 3 portions. Refrigerate if not used immediately and use within 2 weeks or freeze for up to 6 months.

The Ultimate Foot Spa

This is for everyone that has spent one or more days on their feet. This foot bath recipe utilizes one portion of the second extraction of the leftover cannabis bath base maceration.

I include my special essential oil formula here for hot, tired and painful feet, but you can add your own essential oils to make the perfect custom foot bath. I like this bath in a bubbly foot spa or just a basin, either way it's an awesome foot soak that will have you walking on clouds.

Makes 1 foot bath.

You will need:

1/4 cup or 60 grams of coarse Himalayan pink salt, ancient salt, or sea salt

1 portion of the Cannabis Soak Base

2 tbsp or 30 ml of aloe vera gel, scraped from the leaf

1 cup or 240 ml of boiling water and 1 - 2 quarts or 1 - 2 litres of cold, warm or hot water (Your foot bath can be any temperature that you like, including cool, but a cup of boiling water must be added first to aid the mixture in dissolving fully in the water.)

3 drops ginger essential oil

2 drops of peppermint essential oil

2 drops of lemon essential oil

Preparation:

1.   Add the gel from the aloe vera leaf and essential oils to the salt and thoroughly combine.

2.   Add the salt to one portion of the bath base.

3.   Prepare your foot spa or basin with any temperature of water you prefer. Add the foot soak mixture to the water.

Soak for any length of time! This recipe works well in jet foot spas as well as basin soakers.

The Ultimate Hand Plunge

Arthritic hands begone! If you've ever lived with painful and stiff hands, or know someone who does, this hand bath gets right to the pain without any of the psychoactive effects that a full bath may have.

This bath uses a portion of the second extraction and should be made following the same steps as the foot bath. Prepare a deep sink or basin with water as hot as is comfortable for you. You will be soaking your hands for 15 minutes or longer for the most benefit from this hand plunge.

You will need:

1 portion of the Cannabis Soak Base

2 tbsp or 30 ml of aloe vera gel, scraped from the leaf

1 cup or 240 ml of boiling water and enough water to fill the sink and basin

3 drops ginger essential oil

1 drop of ylang ylang essential oil

2 drops of frankincense essential oil

Preparation:

1.   Add the gel from the aloe vera leaf to 1 cup or 240 ml of boiling water and stir. Add the desired essential oils to the cannabis soak base.

2.   Fill a sink or basin with water that is your desired temperature. Add the aloe vera water and the cannabis soak base. Plunge your hands into the water and agitate to dissolve all salts. Continue to soak and massage your hands underwater for 15 minutes or longer.

TIP* I like to reheat the soak water throughout the day and use it multiple times before discarding on those days when my hands need more intensive care. Do this and your hands will thank you!

Chapter 4: Getting Well on Wraps, Masks & Poultices

Cannabis works with wraps, masks and poultices in a way that is similar to lotions and balms. The difference is that it's a more spot-intensive way to use external cannabis and you get the added benefits of detoxifying clay and herbs in these recipes.

Wraps & Poultices

"Poultice" typically means one or more of these techniques: an application of herbal pastes, much like a mask, or an application of herbal teas soaked in gauze or soft hemp fabric and wrapped around a limb or other body part, or a mixture of oils and/or extracts that are applied to an area and covered with cloth bandages or herbs.

Poultices are one of my favorite ways to use cannabis as an herbal medicine. If you don't have time for a cannabis bath, a poultice can be the perfect substitute for the more intensive relief that can be obtained from the baths for joint and muscle pain. Poultices work great for burns and other injuries too.

The Headache Poultice

My favorite way to medicate a nasty headache is with cannabis. There are so many ways to do this, and a cannabis headache poultice ranks right up there, especially when the pain is of the throbbing variety in the front of the head, or due to eye strain.

You will need:

A washcloth or a washcloth size piece of fabric that is very absorbent

1/2 portion of Cannabis Bath Base (Chapter 3)

1 bunch of fresh mint leaves

1 bowl of ice chips

1/2 cup or 120 ml of cold water

Preparation:

1.   Combine the cannabis bath base, mint leaves and a few ice chips in a blender and blend until smooth. Strain the liquid through a cloth bag and add it to a bowl with a few ice chips to keep the liquid cool.

2.   Dip the washcloth into the cold liquid and gently squeeze just enough so it's not "drippy," but still retains much of the liquid. Fold and place over your eyes, forehead or temples. This should remain until the poultice starts to get warm from your body heat, then dip it again in the cold liquid and repeat.

Unused liquid can be frozen in an ice tray, and then used in single portions that are thawed as needed.

Herbal Tea Wrap

Don't have time for a cannabis bath, but need some really intensive relaxation and relief that's fast and also free of any psychoactive effects? Herbal tea poultice wraps really fit the bill!

This wrap uses 1 portion of the cannabis bath base described in Chapter 3. You can make these cannabis bath base portions and freeze them for use in the bath and soak recipes as well as the poultices.

You will need:

Long pieces of gauze, muslin or soft hemp that are clean and dry

Several dry towels for wrapping

1 portion of Cannabis Bath Base (Chapter 3)

1/4 cup or 60 ml fresh aloe vera gel, scraped from the leaf

1/4 cup or 10 grams of chamomile flowers or 10 bags of chamomile tea

1 thumb of ginger, chopped

1 cinnamon stick

2 cups or 480 ml of water

Preparation:

1.   Brew the chamomile flowers, cinnamon and ginger into a very strong tea with the water, and strain.

2.   Add this hot liquid to the aloe vera and cannabis bath base in blender, and then transfer to a pan and gently heat until it is hot, but not hot enough to burn your fingers when you dip the gauze or fabric into the liquid.

3.   Dip the clean pieces of fabric into the liquid and wrap them around sore muscles and joints. Wrap a clean, preferably warm towel around the wet fabric and allow to remain for at least 20 minutes.

Leftover liquid can be refrigerated for no more than 2 weeks. Reheat to the temperature of a cup of tea to repeat the wrap again.

Sunburn Poultice

This is the perfect cooling poultice that draws out heat and promotes healing of the skin.

You will need:

Long pieces of gauze, muslin or soft hemp that are clean and dry

1/4 cup or 60 ml of fresh aloe vera gel, scraped from the leaf

The leftover plant material from making the Cannabis Foundation Oil (Chapter 1)

1/4 cup or 60 ml of orange flower water

1 stalk of fresh lemongrass

1 cup or 240 ml of very cold green tea

Preparation:

1.   In a blender combine the aloe vera, lemongrass stalk, cannabis and orange flower water until smooth and frothy.

2.   Apply this liquid plant paste to the affected areas. Dip the cloth strips in the cold green tea and loosely wrap the areas where the paste has been applied. Leave on for 20 minutes or more, and then remove the paste along with the cloth wrapping. Follow with a cool shower.

Unused paste can be frozen in an ice tray, and then used in single portions that are thawed as needed.

Quick Wrap with Leftover Bath Base Herbs

Got a pile of soapberries and herbs that haven't been extracted a second time yet? You can make a really great therapeutic cannabis wrap!

You will need:

Long pieces of gauze, muslin or soft hemp that are clean and dry

Several dry towels for wrapping

The leftover pulp from making the Cannabis Bath Base (Chapter 3)

2 cups or 480 ml of boiling water

A few drops of any essential oil

Preparation:

1.   Add the boiling water to the leftover pulp. Allow this to stand for 30 minutes and then strain or squeeze through a cloth bag. Add essential oils to the liquid if desired.

2.   You can use this liquid for a hot or cold wrap. Warm or cool the liquid for any application that you choose.

3.   Dip the gauze or other fabric into the liquid and apply to the affected area. You may wrap with a dry and hot towel for a deeper penetration of the healing benefits of this herbal liquid.

Leftover liquid can be refrigerated for no more than 2 weeks.   Reheat to the temperature of a cup of tea to repeat the hot wrap, or use straight from the refrigerator for a cooling wrap.

Apothecary Cannabis Rose Face & Body Mask

Based on the Apothecary Cannabis Rose series of lotions and balms, this face mask uses Ayurvedic herbs such as powdered rose petals and rose water to create a moisturizing (but not greasy) face mask that will minimize fine lines and make your skin as soft and smooth as rose petals.

You will need:

1/2 cup or 70 grams powdered rose petals

2 tbsp or 30 ml Cannabis Foundation Oil (Chapter 1)

2 tbsp or 30 ml fresh aloe vera gel, scraped from the leaf

1/4 cup or 60 ml rose water

1 tsp or 5 ml lemon juice

Preparation:

1.   Combine cannabis oil, olive oil, aloe vera, lemon juice and rose water in a blender. Slowly add the liquid to the powdered rose petals until the consistency is like mashed potatoes.

2.   Apply to face, chest, arms, legs and allow to remain as long as you like; this mask is great for balancing and moisturizing normal to dry skin.

Invigorating Cannabis Citrus Flower Mask

This refreshing mask is great for oily or normal skin. It also doubles as a refresher in hot weather for all skin types!

The special ingredient here, apart from cannabis, is the use of powdered lemon rind, which has exfoliating and regenerating properties. Combined with cannabis, it is an invigorating and healing experience for your skin.

You will need:

1/2 cup or 70 grams powdered lemon rind

2 tbsp or 30 ml Cannabis Foundation Oil (Chapter 1)

2 tbsp or 30 ml fresh aloe vera gel, scraped from the leaf

1/4 cup or 60 ml orange flower water

1 tsp or 5 ml lemon juice

Preparation:

1.   Combine cannabis oil, aloe vera, lemon juice and orange flower water in a blender until smooth and frothy. Slowly add the liquid to the powdered lemon peels until the consistency is like mashed potatoes.

2.   Apply to face, chest, arms, legs (wherever you desire refreshed and renewed skin) for 10 - 15 minutes, and wash off.

Detoxifying Cannabis Clay

This recipe uses any sterilized food-grade mineral clay powder, commonly available at health food stores. This clay is used for both internal and external purposes.

This is also a purifying treatment that is perfect right before one of the cannabis baths in Chapter 3. Apply the clay and allow to dry. Prepare the cannabis bath salts as shown in Chapter 3, and then add to very warm bath water.

You will need:

1/2 cup or 70 grams of sterilized powdered mineral clay

1/4 cup or 60 ml fresh aloe vera gel, scraped from the leaf

2 tbsp or 30 ml Cannabis Foundation Oil (Chapter 1)

1/4 cup or 60 ml very concentrated green tea liquid

1 tsp or 5 ml lemon juice

Preparation:

Combine the aloe vera, green tea, lemon juice and cannabis oil in a blender until smooth and frothy. Slowly add to the powdered clay and mix until creamy. Store in a closed container in the refrigerator for up to 30 days.

Pain Zap Clay

Inspired by the array of spices in my favorite Indo-Pakistani cuisine which are so healing and anti-inflammatory, this pain zapping clay is a favorite.

Do not use on your face or near any mucus membranes because this clay contains spices and herbs that are warm on the skin but extremely hot if you get them in your eyes or mouth. If you do get the clay in your eyes or mouth and it's uncomfortable, rinse your eyes or mouth with regular milk.

This clay is for use on aching backs, swollen joints, swollen feet, etc. Do not use on open wounds. This is the perfect pain relieving treatment to use before taking the Recovery Bath in Chapter 3. After the clay dries, immediately submerge your body in this warm bath; there is no need to wash the clay off ahead of time. This clay can also be used on feet or hands which are then submerged in a full bath, the hand plunge bath, or with a foot spa in Chapter 3.

You will need:

1/2 cup or 70 grams of sterilized powdered mineral clay

3 tbsp or 45 ml Cannabis Foundation Oil (Chapter 1)

1 tbsp or 5 grams powdered turmeric

1 tbsp or 5 grams powdered ginger

Pinch of powdered cloves

Pinch of black pepper powder

Pinch of powdered cinnamon

Pinch of cayenne pepper

1 tsp or 5 ml lemon juice

1/4 cup or 60 ml fresh aloe vera gel, scraped from the leaf

1/4 cup or 60 ml distilled or spring water

Preparation:

Combine the lemon juice, aloe vera, water and cannabis oil in a blender until smooth and frothy. Combine the clay and all powdered spices thoroughly before slowly adding the liquid. Use a hand or stand mixer to whip the mixture until fluffy.

Chapter 5:
Aromatherapy, Tea,
Bhang & Smoothies

Delicious things for your spa day or any day! Try these along with the topicals and baths for a true cannabis spa experience.

Cannabis Aromatherapy

Essence Waters for Glass Service

Living in a legal or medical cannabis state means that you have a lot to choose from! New strains are always being created by growers to express even more flavor in the end product. Cannabis naturally expresses many different flavors through terpene and flavonoid production in the plant itself. I've had cannabis that tasted like lemons, chocolate, spices, oranges, grape soda, mangoes and more.

Cannabis tasting can be as complex as tasting fine wines or cuisine.

Enhancing your cannabis aromatherapy experience is what this chapter is all about.

Smoking is out. It stinks, it's messy and the charred carbon particulates are not good for your lungs. There are two really great ways to enjoy cannabis aromatherapy and each one has its advantages:

1.   A vaporizer - You've probably seen these. They come in box and forced air models usually. They can also be in the form of a pen or other handheld device.

Vaporizers that handle ground flowers are fantastic when you really want to taste all of the flavors the cannabis flower has to offer. Some vaporizers also handle cannabis essential oils and waxes.

2.   A skillet or nail - Vapor bell skillets are relatively new devices that attach to a water pipe. They were originally created to serve "dabs" of essential cannabis oils

and waxes.

But they do more than that. Skillets are also great for vaporizing finely ground cannabis flowers or keif. You can see how clean your vapor actually is by the way your water pipe looks. When you smoke out of a water pipe, the residue left in the pipe is black, charred and tar-like. When you use a skillet, the residue in your water pipe is clean like the residue in a vaporizer, because that's exactly how a vapor bell skillet works: it vaporizes all of the essential oils quickly and cleanly without carbon entering the pipe or your lungs.

Skillets also operate at a higher temperature than a vaporizer. Many people prefer the medicinal effects of cannabinoids that are smoked as opposed to vaped. Skillets produce a vapor that has the same effect as smoked cannabis due to the higher temperatures.

While skillets work beautifully with finely ground cannabis flowers and keif, they do not enhance the flavor experience the way vaporizers do. Cannabis flowers sauteed on a skillet have a more plain and neutral flavor. This is likely due to the very high temperature of the plate.

Your glass bubbler or water pipe can host many different kinds of essential flavors and fragrances in the water, to create a unique aromatherapy experience when you use a vapor bell skillet for cannabis aromatherapy.

What are cannabis essential oils and waxes and how are they used?

Cannabis essential oils and waxes are exactly the kind of flower waxes and essential oils that are produced by the mainstream aromatherapy industry, using identical chemistry, and in many cases the same techniques, to produce a high quality essential oil product.

Cannabis essential oils can be 70% or higher in THC.

Taking a cue from the mainstream aromatherapy industry where CO_2 has become quite popular, many cannabis dispensaries now offer CO_2 extracted oils. The cannabis oils retain the lovely flavonoids and terpenes along with the medicinal cannabinoids. This eco-friendly and healthier form of extraction produces a superior cannabis essential oil in every way.

Flower & Fruit Essence Technique for Your Bubbler

Essence waters are a "living" water made with fresh flowers, herbs and fruits as opposed to distilled floral hydrosols like rose water or orange flower water.

The technique for creating a whole living water essence is simple and has been used for hundreds of years. An example of the living water essence technique is the Bach Flower Remedy. The technique in this book differs from the Bach method in that it's not a homeopathic dilution, and instead contains the full aroma and taste of the flowers, herbs and fruits that are used to make the water.

You will need:

Any combination of fresh flowers, herbs or fruit. My favorite combination is sliced oranges and fresh roses.

A glass bowl filled with spring or purified water.

A sunny day outside or a warm sunny indoor windowsill. I prefer a windowsill indoors that gets a few hours of direct sun.

A small mesh filter or screen that won't block sunlight to keep out debris and insects if you are putting the bowl outside to extract.

Preparation:

1.   Place all of the plant material in the bowl, and press down the plant material a few times to gently bruise the material so it will begin to release essential flavors and fragrances. Pour water over the plant material until the water completely covers it. You may add stone weights if necessary to keep the plant material submerged. Put in a very warm and sunny place for 3 hours or more.

2.   Strain the plant material from the essence water and store in the refrigerator for up to a week. It's ready to use in your bubbler as soon as it is strained, but it is even more delicious when chilled first!

Bubbler Aromatherapy With Floral and Herbal Hydrosol

Another way to enjoy an aromatherapeutic experience with your bubbler is with commercially available floral and herbal water, or hydrosol. These are commonly available in ethnic grocers or natural food stores. Some of the more common varieties of these are rose water, orange flower water and mint water. Choose one that does not contain preservatives and keep it refrigerated when not in use.

Add 1 part of hydrosol to 5 parts of plain water for a more intense flavor and aroma.

Drop this down 1 to 10 or greater dilution for more subtle effects.

If your bubbler has ice pinches, use them. Ice and chilled water enhance the experience even more!

Tea, Bhang and Smoothies

No spa day is complete without refreshing beverages!

Some of these recipes do contain cannabis and therefore THC, as noted in each recipe. Please plan your activities accordingly, and avoid operating heavy machinery or driving.

Apothecary Cannabis Rose Chai

A sublime chai that you will fall in love with; this is a rose garden in a tea cup.

I've always dreamed of growing cannabis in a rose garden, and this lovely chai is as close as I've come to capturing that dream in a single recipe. I hope you'll love it as much as I do!

Makes 4 servings. *Contains THC

You will need:

1 tbsp or 1 gram of rose petals

1 tbsp or 2 grams of black tea

1 green cardamom pod

1 cinnamon stick

1 tbsp or 5 grams of demerara or other natural sugar

1/4 cup or 60 grams of shelled raw hemp seed

1/4 cup or 60 ml rose water

1 gram or more of potent cannabis flowers, finely ground

1 tbsp or 15 ml of coconut oil or grass-fed ghee

2 cups or 480 ml of water

Preparation:

1.   Prepare 2 pans on the stove. One that will contain the tea ingredients, and the other that will contain the cannabis milk.

2.   In the first pan for the tea, put 1 cup or 240 ml of water in the pan along with the rose petals, black tea, broken cardamom pod and cinnamon stick. Heat this until it boils, and remove from the heat and allow to steep while preparing the cannabis milk.

3.   In the second pan, heat the cannabis and oil on low for 10 minutes.

4.   In the blender add 1 cup or 240 ml of water, hemp seed, sugar and blend until milky. Add this to the cannabis and oil in the pan and stir frequently, holding the temperature around 300 F or 150 C for 5 minutes. Remove from the heat.

5.   Add the rose water to the pan with the warm tea ingredients, and then strain the tea into individual cups. Follow by straining the cannabis milk evenly into each cup. Add more hot water as needed to fill the cups, and serve.

Soothing Tummy Bhang

This bhang recipe is so simple, yet so effective for upset tummies! Ginger is featured prominently in this recipe, and I recommend that you get it fresh and slice or shred it yourself for the best results.

Makes 4 servings. *Contains THC

You will need:

1/2 cup or 100 grams of thinly sliced or shredded fresh ginger root

1/4 cup or 60 grams of shelled raw hemp seed

1 gram or more of potent cannabis flowers, finely ground

1 tbsp or 15 ml of coconut oil or grass-fed ghee

2 cups or 480 ml of water

1 tbsp or 5 grams of demerara or natural sugar

Preparation:

1.   Prepare 2 pans on the stove. One that will contain the ginger tea, and the other that will contain the cannabis milk.

2.   In the first pan for the tea, put 1 cup or 240 ml of water in the pan along with the sliced or shredded ginger and sugar. Heat this until it boils and remove from the heat and allow to steep while preparing the cannabis milk.

3.   In the second pan, heat the cannabis and oil on low for 10 minutes.

4.   In the blender add 1 cup or 240 ml of water, hemp seed, sugar and blend until milky. Add this to the cannabis

and oil in the pan and stir frequently holding the temperature around 300 F or 150 C for 5 minutes. Remove from the heat.

5.   Strain the ginger tea into each cup. Strain the cannabis milk evenly into each cup and top with enough hot water to fill the cups, and serve.

European Cannabis Sipping Chocolate

A thick, dark chocolate drink that is perfect for holiday entertaining or any time. Float fresh raspberries on the finished chocolate or dust with cinnamon for the finishing touch.

Makes 4 servings. *Contains THC

You will need:

3 tbsp or 15 grams of raw powdered cacao

1 tsp or 5 ml of vanilla extract

3 tbsp or 45 grams of demerara or natural sugar

1/3 cup shelled raw hemp seed

1 tbsp or 15 ml of coconut oil or grass-fed ghee

1 gram or more of potent cannabis flowers, finely ground

2 cups or 480 ml of water

Preparation:

1.   In a pan on the stove, heat the cannabis and the oil on low heat for 10 minutes.

2.   In a blender, combine the water, hemp seed, cacao, vanilla and sugar until smooth.

3.   Return the pan with the cannabis and oil to the stove and pour in the hemp chocolate mixture. Heat this to 300 F or 150 C for about 5 minutes. Serve immediately in small European-style chocolate cups.

Blood Orange Hemp Cream Smoothie

Another wintry favorite that's perfect for the holidays or Valentine's Day. Its pretty pink color comes from the blood orange, which has a berry-orange flavor that is totally unique to this variety of orange. It's packed with 10 grams of protein per serving too!

Makes 4 servings. *Does NOT contain THC

You will need:

1 quart or 1 litre of freshly squeezed blood orange juice

2 large bananas

2 tsp or 10 ml vanilla extract

1/2 cup or 125 grams of ice chips or cubes

1 cup or 250 grams of shelled raw hemp seed

Preparation:

Everything goes straight into the blender and is blended until creamy and smooth. Serve immediately.

Mango Hemp Lassi

It is thought that mango potentiates the effects of cannabis, which makes this the perfect smoothie to enjoy while soaking in a cannabis bath or after massaging in a topical lotion or balm.

This mango lassi is vegan and has 10 grams of protein per serving.

Makes 4 servings. *Does NOT contain THC

You will need:

2 large or 4 small mangoes, peeled and sliced

1 cup or 250 grams of shelled raw hemp seed

1 tsp or 5 ml of vanilla extract

1 cup or 240 ml chilled water

1 cup or 250 grams of ice chips or cubes

1 dash of black salt (This is optional, but very good and the secret to a great mango lassi!)

1 dash of cinnamon

Preparation:

Everything goes straight into the blender and is blended until creamy and smooth. Serve immediately.

Hemp New York Egg Cream

A classic fountain favorite - the New York Egg Cream is loved by grown-ups and kids everywhere!

This version has a wealth of protein and nutrients, which makes it a really smart sweet treat or snack any time.

Makes 4 servings. *Does NOT contain THC

You will need:

3 tbsp or 15 grams of raw cacao powder

1 tbsp or 15 ml vanilla extract

1 cup or 250 grams of shelled raw hemp seed

1/4 cup or 60 grams of demerara or natural sugar

2 cups or 480 ml of chilled seltzer or sparkling water

1 cup or 250 grams of ice chips or cubes

Preparation:

Put everything into the blender until it becomes a frothy milk with a "head." Pour into glasses and serve with a straw!

Conclusion & Resource Guide

I've included my favorite ingredient and tool resources for making every recipe in this book in this section. Nothing in this section is a paid endorsement - these are brands and shops that I personally patronize, as I am pleased with the quality of ingredients they carry.

Natural Foods Stores and Amazon.com

Hands down the best two places to find almost every ingredient or tool you will need to make the recipes in this book.

Natur-Oli Soapberries - naturoli.com

My favorite brand of soapberry, and the one I use for making the cannabis bath bases. They also sell their soapberries on Amazon, but they often have great deals in their own online shop, so check that out too. Their soapberries are very fresh and organic.

Camden Grey - camdengrey.com

Some of the more exotic recipes in this book use rare and luxurious ingredients, like floral waxes, essential flower oils and tropical butters. Camden Grey is a well-respected source for these precious ingredients at a surprisingly reasonable price! They also have great customer service, and include free gifts of new essential oil samples and other kinds of ingredient samples in each order.

Your Local Ethnic Supermarket

Many of the recipes in this book use ingredients that are quite common in ethnic Indian and Middle Eastern supermarkets, including oils, spices and fresh herbs.

Mehandi Henna - Mehandi.com

The only online store where I have been able to find real henna flower essential oil. A $10 vial will make many recipes in this book!

Recipe Index

- mango seed butter
- tucuma or murumuru butter
- jasmine floral wax
- ginger essential oil
- true ceylon cinnamon
  essential oil
- soap candy molds

4 oz /$5 /lb
16 oz /lb

13086466R00084

Made in the USA
San Bernardino, CA
08 July 2014